# Let Him Not Sink

**Dr Samir Parikh** is an eminent psychiatrist working in the field of mental health over the past two decades. He is currently the Director of the Department of Mental Health and Behavioural Sciences at Fortis Healthcare and is also the Chairperson of the Fortis National Mental Health Council, Fortis National Mental Health Program. Under his guidance and leadership the Department of Mental Health and Behavioural Sciences works to provide comprehensive mental health services and also conducts specialized programs for the community. These include the Fortis School Mental Health Program, Fortis Organizational Psychology Initiative and the Fortis Community Outreach Program. Dr Parikh has conducted various studies that have been published in the media that has helped the community get an insight into mental health issues.

**Kamna Chhibber** is an eminent clinical psychologist. She is currently the Head of Mental Health for the Fortis National Mental Health Program and also heads the Department of Mental Health and Behavioural Sciences at Fortis Healthcare. Ms Chhibber is a trained Cognitive Behaviour Therapist who works within an eclectic frame for the treatment of clinical and other related problems in children, adolescents and adults. With an experience over a decade in the field of mental health, she has been instrumental in the development and shaping of the Fortis School Mental Health Program. Ms Chhibber has been working extensively with schools, students, teachers, parents, as well as within the community towards making mental health a talking point and a priority for all.

# Let Him Not Sink
## First Steps to Mental Health

A Manual for Adults who Work Closely
with Children and Adolescents

## Samir Parikh
### & Kamna Chhibber

Published by
Rupa Publications India Pvt. Ltd 2017
7/16, Ansari Road, Daryaganj
New Delhi 110002

*Sales centres:*
Allahabad Bengaluru Chennai
Hyderabad Jaipur Kathmandu
Kolkata Mumbai

copyright © Samir Parikh & Kamna Chhibber 2017

The views and opinions expressed in this book are the author's own and the facts are as reported by him which have been verified to the extent possible, and the publishers are not in any way liable for the same.
All rights reserved.

No part of this publication may be reproduced, transmitted, or stored in a retrieval system, in any form or by any means, electronic, mechanical, photocopying, recording or otherwise, without the prior permission of the publisher.

ISBN: 978-81-291-4887-2

First impression 2017

10 9 8 7 6 5 4 3 2 1

Printed at Replika Press Pvt. Ltd.

This book is sold subject to the condition that it shall not, by way of trade or otherwise, be lent, resold, hired out, or otherwise circulated, without the publisher's prior consent, in any form of binding or cover other than that in which it is published.

# CONTENTS

*Contributors* — vii

*Preface* — ix

Introduction: First Steps to Mental Health — 1

1. The Problem Areas — 6
2. Understanding Mental Health and Related Illnesses — 9
3. Essential Skills for Working with Children and Adolescents — 14
4. Depression — 23
5. Bipolar and Related Disorders — 34
6. Anxiety Disorders — 47
7. Separation Anxiety — 61
8. Selective Mutism — 69
9. Obsessive-Compulsive Disorder — 78
10. Somatic Symptoms and Related Disorders — 90
11. Attention-Deficit/Hyperactivity Disorder — 101
12. Disruptive Behaviour Disorders — 113
13. Eating Disorders — 127

| | |
|---|---|
| 14. Substance Use Disorders | 140 |
| 15. Schizophrenia in Children and Adolescents | 154 |
| 16. Intellectual Disability | 167 |
| 17. Specific Learning Disability | 179 |
| 18. Autism Spectrum Disorder | 192 |
| 19. Trauma and Abuse | 202 |
| 20. Suicide and Self-Harm | 215 |
| *Fortis Healthcare Limited* | 228 |
| *Fortis School Mental Health Program* | 228 |
| *References* | 230 |

**Key Contributors:**
Mimansa Singh
Divya Jain
Roshni Sondhi

**Contributors:**
Chitwan Singh
Pratishtha Trivedi
Kanika Mehrotra
Geetika Virdi
Pallavi Sharma
Hargun Ahluwalia
Kanika Soni
Hina Zutshi

# PREFACE

After working in the sector of schoolchildren's mental health for over two decades one recognizes the various vectors—psychological, social, behavioural and environmental—that affect the lives of students making it imperative for people like me to work with them and all those having an impact on their lives—parents, teachers and support staff. Students do experience significant stress at times, which makes it necessary for us to focus on their behavioural and emotional health, equipping them with the right skills to lead a healthy life.

Research has highlighted the need to place impetus on the collaboration between schools and outside agencies that work in the domain of child and adolescent health and well-being. This has highlighted to me the need for school-linked services which lay emphasis on training, early identification, promotion of positive social and emotional development and as a result early intervention for all mental health-related concerns for students.

Equipping adults who work in the school system with the right knowledge and requisite skills is the correct next step. It's for this purpose that *Let Him Not Sink* has been written to act as a guide for adults working with children facilitating early identification, providing key signs and symptoms pertaining to various clinical conditions and also the effective first steps to working on the problem.

Nothing can substitute early intervention in order to tackle mental health issues. Before such issues swell up to a level where it becomes resistant to treatment, we need to be able to reach out to those who need help.

Samir Parikh<br>
August, 2017

# Introduction

# FIRST STEPS TO MENTAL HEALTH

### What is Mental Health?[1]

World Health Organization defines **mental health** as a 'state of well-being in which every individual realizes his own potential, can cope with the normal stresses of life, can work productively and fruitfully, and is able to make a contribution to his community.' In the context of children and adolescents this would imply the ability to forge relationships, perform academically, display appropriate behaviour, have control over their thought processes and be in charge of their emotional experiences.

Anyone might have issues regarding their mental health. But these translate into being called an **illness** only when they significantly compromise the daily functioning of the individual, impacting moods, thoughts and behaviour, causing an alteration in relatedness and the ability to engage with their daily routine.

### Facts about mental health problems

- **Children and adolescents can have mental illnesses**

---

[1] Mental health and concepts related to it are discussed in greater detail in chapter 2 of the book.

It is a fact that children and adolescents too can have mental health concerns. How they express it can be different from the way adults do, which is one of the factors that makes it even more difficult to identify and treat these issues.

If you work with children every day then you might have come across children with behavioural concerns or those displaying cognitive and emotional deficits. It could be something as basic as an inability to concentrate on tasks or instances of truant and disruptive behaviour. More often than not these behavioural problems could be an indication of mental health problems. These can include depression, anxiety, substance use disorder or attention-deficit/hyperactivity disorder and autism spectrum disorders, to name a few.

These disorders can begin in childhood or adolescence and if left untreated they can strengthen over time, easily progressing into more severe forms. Many a times correct identification or intervention does not happen as the adults associated with the child's life are unaware of the signs and symptoms of these conditions and what the first-steps are to providing appropriate care. Correct and timely identification, diagnosis and intervention can ensure that the children grow up to be healthy, happy and responsible adult members of the society.

- **Stigma and misinformation are abundantly attached to mental health illness**

Due to lack of awareness, mental health illnesses are shrouded in stigma and misconception. This stigma is the reason why individuals and families frequently turn a blind eye to potential mental health problems and do not seek the much required help.

Challenges also arise on account of individual factors. A child or an adolescent may be reluctant to discuss his problems with another person. He or she might worry about being misjudged, not being understood or feel their confidence might be betrayed, thereby experiencing mistrust and shame. They might not know who to ask for help, or might be misinformed about the nature of their problem. Often they may not even be aware that they have a problem and can carry the agonizing pain of feeling responsible for their own suffering, experiencing a lot of guilt and self-blame. This can be further compounded by the lack of understanding and awareness amongst parents and other members of the community.

As parents, teachers, counsellors and community workers it is important that you help the community develop a greater understanding of mental health illness, the treatments available for it, know the people who can offer the right assistance, and most importantly—spread the message that mental health problems are treatable and can be managed with the right help and support.

- **Dealing with a mental health crisis requires knowledge and understanding**

A **mental health crisis** refers to any situation occurring on account of a mental health illness that puts the child or others around him at any such risk which even the adults are unable to handle with the given resources. **Mental health crises can occur as a result of acute changes in the child or adolescent which can reflect in terms of their thoughts, emotions or behaviour.** It can occur without any warning and it is as important to be able to deal with it as it is to deal with any physical health crisis. This includes understanding the signs of a mental health problem, utilizing strategies to de-escalate the crisis and formulating a crisis management plan while enlisting the right kind of support for the child.

## Why do you need First Steps to Mental Health (FSMH)?

If you are involved with children and adolescents, it is essential to be equipped to handle challenges regarding mental health. Close to 15 million individuals are battling with some or the other form of mental health illness in India. 10 per cent of all children suffer from some form of mental health issue and more than 50 per cent of these go untreated and many more undetected (Medindia, 2010). This book aims to serve as an interface between mental health professionals and those working in close association with children, enabling better identification of such illnesses and concerns in order to provide the right professional help to those in need.

We hope to provide you with the right tools and strategies for primary intervention—including identifying the children at risk, provision of initial care and support, and guidance for generating appropriate help that is specific to our culture keeping in mind the challenges it poses.

*Let Him Not Sink* hopes to empower you. Our work as mental health professionals working in a multi-disciplinary team, including psychiatrists, clinical psychologists, counselling psychologists, psycho-analysts, psychodynamic psychotherapists, art therapists, special educators and occupational therapists, has time and again reacquainted us with the need for clear and cogent information on mental health illnesses. Having the knowledge of how to work with an individual who has been identified with an illness is crucial. Lack of information and guidance is often the cause of conditions going unrecognized, lack of timely help being provided and an inability for an adult to reach out to a child at risk. **To be informed is to be empowered and that is the aim towards which this book is directed.**

We are confident that this book will serve as a useful source of information and provide the guidance to help you help the children you come in contact with.

It is important to be equipped to handle adverse situations arising out of mental health problems and providing the child or adolescent with the kind of support that he requires depending on the type and severity of the crisis. Being trained in the first steps to mental health will enable you to identify a problem and provide initial intervention, which is a key to determining how quickly the child will receive the right kind of assistance.

# 1
# THE PROBLEM AREAS

This book is designed to give you first-hand, practical information on how to deal with problems regarding mental health that you may encounter while working with children and adolescents in quick, easy steps. The book provides a step-by-step primary care intervention for common mental health conditions and developmental disorders found in children and adolescents, equipping you to apply these steps to take care of problems at the grass roots level in a bid to create an atmosphere of self-sufficiency.

We will be focussing on the following issues:

1. Depression
2. Bipolar and related disorders
3. Anxiety disorders
    - Generalized anxiety disorder
    - Panic disorder
    - Phobia
4. Separation anxiety disorders
5. Selective mutism
6. Obsessive-compulsive disorder
7. Somatic symptom disorder
8. Attention-deficit/hyperactivity disorder
9. Disruptive behaviour disorders

- Oppositional defiant disorder
- Conduct disorder
10. Eating disorders
    - Anorexia nervosa
    - Bulimia nervosa
11. Substance abuse
12. Schizophrenia
13. Intellectual disability
14. Learning disability
15. Autism spectrum disorders
16. Trauma and abuse
17. Suicide and self-harm

The aim of getting this book published is to enable you, the adult in direct contact with the affected children and adolescents, to provide the initial care and support and guide them to the right professional help, if required, for a range of disorders and mental health problems. It also hopes to, through you, reduce the stigma associated with such illnesses in the community at large.

## The FSMH steps

When we look at any challenge related to mental health or issue being faced by a child or an adolescent, there are six primary steps to ensuring that the child is able to cope, moving beyond the challenges posed by the illness to lead a fulfilling and productive life unhindered by any mental health problem. Each of these steps forms an integral part of the primary intervention that should be implemented by you and the book highlights how these steps should be implemented in specific ways with regards to specific mental health conditions. In conditions where these exact steps may not be applicable we have provided you with alternate modalities of working with the child and his family.

### The First Steps to Mental Health

**Step 1** – Identify the children at risk
**Step 2** – Evaluate the degree of risk to self and to others
**Step 3** – Listen non-judgementally and give reassurance
**Step 4** – Inform the caregiver when required and if available
**Step 5** – Encourage help-seeking and provide information
**Step 6** – Build resilience post-intervention

This six-step action plan is designed to enable you to recognize, manage and support those experiencing any of the mental health and developmental disorders discussed in the book. According to the nature of the disorder or the need of the situation, it is possible that the order of the steps may vary while some may be omitted or others may be added. For example, while it is of undeniable importance that risk for suicide is assessed, you may need to first provide a non-judgemental listening ear to help the child talk about the problem.

Frequently, problems can go undetected as children may not know whom to turn to for help. Children in emotional distress need to be heard, without their concerns being dismissed. They might be feeling betrayed, judged, troubled, lonely and unaccepted and need understanding and reassurance before they are open to guidance and direction from you.

In any crisis, it is important that the intervention provider ensures safety of himself and others. Usually during a mental health crisis the person in question is in danger of harming himself as opposed to others. The person providing FSMH should be flexible and responsive. He should be able to use his own judgement with regard to which step is needed at what point.

This book is not meant to be a diagnostic tool or a guide to take the place of a mental health professional. It is a handbook to help the adult in the situation, provide primary intervention to the child till the right help is availed.

# 2
# UNDERSTANDING MENTAL HEALTH AND RELATED ILLNESSES

## What is mental health?

According to the WHO, 'Health is a state of complete physical, mental and social well-being and not merely the absence of disease or infirmity.' When a person is in a state of mental well-being or is mentally healthy, he can cope with his life roles and responsibilities and is aware of his strengths. A child with a healthy mind has the capability to think clearly and logically, enjoy healthy relationships with parents, teachers and friends and feel a sense of happiness and confidence in his abilities.

A mentally healthy child is happy and interactive at an individual, peer, family, school and community level. The importance of mental health in the quality of life of an individual is significantly under-recognized in our country. Mental health is imperative in ensuring social and emotional well-being and is crucial in the development of adequate coping resources that help an individual effectively face the challenges of life. Prevention and intervention of any related illness at an early stage can help transform at-risk children into healthy and contributing adults of society.

As the adults who work closely with children, we must understand the importance of ensuring the mental health and well-being of children by learning to identify and deal with situations in which the child's mental health has been compromised as well as working on preventive measures to promote positive mental health and well-being.

## What is mental health illness?

The absence of mental health can lead to mental health illnesses. Very simply, a mental health illness can be defined as a set of cognitive, behavioural or emotional states that deviate from the idea of what is 'normal'. These conditions tend to occur with a frequency, intensity and duration that cause disruption in a person's day-to-day social and occupational functioning.

A mental health disorder causes significant maladaptive changes in a person's thinking patterns, emotional experiences and behavioural responses which impact their ability to study, concentrate and engage effectively in interpersonal relationships. Different mental health disorders have different prevalence rates. However, the impact they have upon an individual tends to be significant as it impairs the emotional, social and occupational functioning of the person. In the context of children this would imply the inability to participate in social interactions, deterioration in academic performance, reduction in play and fun activities and increase in irritability or anger, to name a few.

Mental health illnesses might seem intimidating, especially if you have not had any prior experience in knowing, understanding or working with them. It is important to remember that regardless of the nature of the illness, it causes a lot of pain and suffering to the individual and the family alike. This problem is often magnified in children as they are not as equipped as adults are to deal with difficult emotions, being able to identify them or knowing effective coping strategies to handle them. Children's lack of a comprehensive vocabulary to be able to describe their experiences further contributes to the challenge posed by the situation.

## What causes mental health illnesses?

The onset of a mental health illness is typically the result of the interplay of two or more dynamic factors in a person that finally precipitates a breakdown in the form of such an illness. These factors include:

- *Biological factors*

    Mental health disorders have a significant biochemical component. Research has shown that when the levels of certain neurotransmitters (natural chemicals in the brain that send messages to nerve-cells or neurons) in the brain go through an abnormal increase or decrease it leads to the precipitation of a mental health illness.

- *Genetic factors*

    Mental health disorders, especially developmental disorders, have a strong genetic component associated with them. Such illnesses often have a family history. This is seen as an important risk factor in the aetiology of mental health illnesses.

- *Environmental factors*

    Sometimes a child can be the victim of hostile environmental conditions such as a traumatic event, dysfunctional family relationships and abuse, to name a few. Lack of nurturance, consistency and security in the environment can lead to the development of deficient coping strategies in the child making him vulnerable to mental health illnesses.

## How is a mental health illness treated?

- *Psychiatric medications*

    Medications that are safe and effective and can be given to children and adolescents are available, making treatment and management of mental health illnesses more efficacious. Such medications can be prescribed only by a psychiatrist. There can be situations in which a child may need to be hospitalized such as in cases of acute psychosis, aggression and violence, or in the case of substance abuse and suicidality. Often parents, caregivers and we as professionals in the field tend to have misgivings about medications and its effects anticipating that they may be addictive and could have extreme side effects. It is important to remember that these fears are usually unfounded and that parents/caregivers should be encouraged to discuss their doubts and queries with the mental health professional treating their child.

- *Psychotherapy and supportive services*

    Psychotropic medication is only one of the steps to effective treatment. Often psychotherapy is required to take care of the child's emotional and social aspects of well-being. These psychotherapeutic interventions are required for the individual and sometimes can also include the family in what is called family psychotherapy. Interventions can be provided in both an individual as well as a group setting. In certain developmental disorders like autism, or learning disabilities, other specialized service providers may also be required like a special educator, occupational therapist, or rehabilitation services through a trained psychologist.

- *Community support*

    Effective reintegration into the community following treatment is necessary for any child who has had a mental health illness. This is the collective responsibility of the family, teachers, counsellors or the community workers who are associated with the child. Your role starts with enabling early identification to assist in effective reintegration of the child through acceptance, social support and building the child's resilience.

# 3
# ESSENTIAL SKILLS FOR WORKING WITH CHILDREN AND ADOLESCENTS

Before we enter into the space of specific clinical syndromes and conditions, it is important to look at the basic skills you need to be empowered with and have knowledge of as you enter into the environment of the place you work in. The two most important people you would be dealing with would be the parent or caregiver and the child who is at risk or already has a problem. Being able to approach both of them is the first step and there are some things you would need to keep in mind before you do so. Let's take a look at what these things are which form the basis of the communication and interaction you would be having with them.

## Talking to the parent/caregiver about the problem

One of the first and probably the most important step in dealing with a mental health illness or a crisis is informing the parent or caregiver about the problem and directing them to the right kind of support services. This can be a very challenging step for you as you may be faced with different reactions from the parent. These can vary from ignorance to anger and denial or even self-blame and criticalness towards the self. You might find yourself in a situation where there might not be a responsible adult to inform, especially if you are a community worker and might be directly responsible for getting the child the right kind of help.

When you are breaking the news to a parent, it is important for you to be able to communicate your understanding of the parents' situation and that you are working towards the same end, namely, the well-being of the child or adolescent concerned. It can be very difficult for a parent to accept that their child may have a problem. Understanding a parent's perspective can go a long way in securing his or her cooperation in developing and implementing an effective intervention for the child.

## Breaking the news:

- **Talk about the problem in a sensitive, blame-free manner.** The way the parent or caregiver first hears and understands the problem defines the way in which he looks at the condition and the effects it will have on the future prospects of their child. The kind of hope that is instilled in the parent at this stage will pave the way forward for his attitude towards the child, his illness and the professionals they will come in contact with in the future.
- **Try and determine the level of acceptance the parent has about the problem.** You can actively work on this by eliciting the problems they might have observed in the child at home in a sympathetic manner. Once these problems are listed you can join the dots and explain why you feel the child may require professional help. Helping a parent make sense of the problems in a coherent manner is the right step towards building acceptance.
- **Share your concerns** about the child and the behaviour displayed by him that you feel might be problematic. Do so

in a blame-free and calm manner. Do not label the child and do not diagnose. It is best to talk in the form of observable behaviour that they too will be able to identify with.

- **Understand their anxieties and fears** and encourage them to ask questions and share their concerns. The more they will know and understand the problem, the more you will be able to enlist their cooperation in dealing with the situations that would present themselves in the future.
- **Reflect their feelings** of hurt, shock, disappointment, anger, sadness and even guilt and convey to them that you understand this might be something which is difficult to accept and adjust to. Explain them the importance of their acceptance and support to be able to provide the right help to the child as early as possible.
- **Instil hope** by sharing with them the efficacy and effectiveness of treatments that are available for the problems being observed. Drawing parallels with physical health conditions can make the problem more relatable for the parent and enable them to maintain hopefulness.
- **Do your homework.** Make sure you are able to tell the parent what the next step is and refer them to the right professional. If you are bombarded with questions about the condition that you may feel ill-equipped to answer make sure that you readily admit to all that you don't know and encourage them to clarify their doubts with a professional.

**Concerns parents may have:**

It is important to understand the basic worries, apprehensions and concerns of a parent in order to effectively address them. As someone working closely with children and adolescents, you often may have to take on the role of the **advocate in favour of the child's mental health**. Understanding the parents' concerns enables you and them to form a partnership to ensure the effective development of the child.

- **Unfulfilled expectations**

  All parents have some dreams about their children and their future achievements and it can be very hard to accept the child's limitations and face the reality that he might not be like other children or may not be able to achieve up to his full potential. It is important to help them normalize the issue and offer them hope and the possibilities of treatment.

- **Stigma in society**

  Mental health illness has a stigma associated with it and knowing that your child might be suffering from it may be difficult to accept. Parents might worry about how other children and parents will treat their child. Social exclusion due to a mental health illness can be a very significant and unfortunate reality. Parents may also feel that others may not be sensitive to the needs of their child.

- **Friendships compromised**

  All parents want their children to have friends. Parents of children with mental health illness will be especially sensitive about their child's ability to make and keep friends. It is important to break down certain myths and information barriers within the school or the community that are obstacles to these children being rehabilitated and reintegrated into spaces formerly occupied by them.

- **Self-blame**

  Not many parents understand the concept of mental health illnesses. It can seem fear-inducing and inexplicable to many. In such a scenario many parents wonder if they have made mistakes in their upbringing to induce the problem in their child. Providing correct information to the parent, therefore, becomes crucial to combat the problem of self-blame, criticalness and guilt.

- **Lack of guidance**

    Many parents feel like they don't know how to deal with the challenge posed by the problem. They don't know where to go for help and the lack of awareness makes them susceptible to many myths about the illness. They can be confused as to how to deal with it or even how to recognize it. They can have many doubts about how to parent the child now that a problem has been identified.

**Talking to the child at risk**

Given your role and position in the child's life, you will be one of the first people to notice and be approached by a child at risk. These communications can be complex and sensitive and can also pave the way for future decision-making for the child or adolescent. It is important to be aware of certain skills to help you talk about the problem in the right manner, handle the child's distress and direct them towards the right help.

It is important to communicate to the child that you are there to help and that he does not need to continue facing the problem alone. Offer him your support and inform about the next steps towards the right help. Once the child feels heard and accepted, he will be open to and trusting of your guidance. Without really listening to the child's problems, referring the child or his parents for further help may actually prove to be fruitless. Certain basic but essential skills to keep in mind include the following:

- **Listen**

    An important aspect of active listening is never to assume that you know what the person is going through, but rather to make an honest effort to understand his subjective experience. When talking to a child or an adolescent, sit or crouch at the child's eye level—it helps in forming a rapport with the child. Pay attention to the non-verbal signs as well. In order to truly make an impact or connect effectively it is important that you refrain from giving advice at each step. Do not interrupt the child and keep in mind that this could be his first opportunity to be heard. Provide a non-threatening and safe environment to enable him to talk about his problem.

- **Reassure**

    When a child comes to you with a problem, or you approach a child with certain concerns it is natural that the child may be hesitant to share his troubles with you. Reassure him and give him positive feedback for coming to seek help or recognizing that there is a problem and wanting to find a solution to it. Many children might come to you as a last resort or when they feel they have no options left. In this case it becomes very important to provide them hope for the future and an assurance of support and guidance. Give the child time and space to be able to talk about his problem. Don't be impatient as it can take multiple interactions with the child to break the ice and bridge the gap.

- **Reflect**

    When talking to a child or an adolescent you should try and talk in a language that he is comfortable with. Encourage them to talk about their concerns and feelings. Do not be judgemental. Be aware that you might be coming from an entirely different value-system in comparison to the child. This difference can often come in the way of connecting with the child. In such instances, bring the focus back to the child's distress and suffering. Enable the child to label his feelings and emotions. These words need to be such that children can identify with them—angry, sad and scared, to name a few. Do not catastrophize by using extreme words such as 'devastating', 'terrible' or 'horrible'. Reflecting feelings can also serve as a self-check loop.

- **Empathize**

  Empathy quite simply refers to the ability to step into another person's shoes and understand the situation from his point of view. Asking open-ended questions, clarifying with the child what he is feeling are all tools to develop an empathetic listening. It is important to ask the child about concrete details, with vivid and rich explanations and then summarizing succinctly what the child has told you in simple language. Empathy is not to be confused with sympathy. It doesn't involve feeling sorry for the person or pitying them. It refers to understanding the experience of the other person and respecting them as individuals with their unique strengths and weaknesses.

- **Use the child's language**

  Children below the age of twelve do not understand abstract concepts and it is important to use direct and easy language when communicating with them. The use of metaphors like stories, fictional characters and poems is very useful in helping the child form a rapport and build trust in you. The use of play is also a helpful tool when talking with children as they don't always express themselves in words like adults. Adolescents and teenagers prefer to be spoken to like adults; they might perceive you to be condescending if you try to address their concerns or feelings in a child-like way. It is important to gauge the situation and modify the methods you use to talk to the child accordingly.

- **Maintain boundaries**

  An important aspect of being in the helping role, especially with children and adolescents is drawing the line. It is natural to want to protect and rescue the children at risk as we get in touch with their vulnerability and helplessness. However, it is very important to understand your role and the limitations that come with it. Stepping out of your boundaries and trying to take on more than your own role in the life of the child can lead to many complications and detrimental consequences such as burnout and dependency issues. Sometimes the child or the parents can be overbearing, placing excessive demands on you and in these cases it is imperative to set certain rules and limits that should not be crossed. For instance, talking or reaching out to you at a specific time only during the day.

- **Guide**

  If you listen to the child empathically and non-judgementally, you will have built a healthy rapport and would be in a clearer position to gauge the situation. By talking to the child about his problem, you should have answers to the following questions:
  - Is this a mental health crisis?
  - Who needs to be informed? (Parent/caregiver/resource-person within the community or organization)

- Does the child need to be referred to a mental health professional? (psychiatrist/psychologist)

Once you have clarity on the situation and its severity, you will be able to correctly guide the child towards adequate and timely intervention.

| Dos and Don'ts that You Should Keep in Mind ||
|---|---|
| Dos | Don'ts |
| Listen empathetically | Force the child to talk |
| Provide reassurance | Be judgemental |
| Assess if the situation is a crisis | Interrupt the child |
| Talk in simple and clear language | Give advice |
| Ask open-ended questions | Talk too much |
| Reflect feelings | Try to solve the problem on your own |
| Paraphrase and clarify | Label |
| Encourage child to label his emotions | Patronize or focus on the child's weakness |
| Use relatable metaphors | |
| Listen more and talk less | |
| Guide and refer to the right help | |
| Focus on strengths | |
| Refer to an expert where required | |

# 4
# DEPRESSION[2]

We all feel sad or low, which we frequently label as being 'depressed', at some time or the other in our lives. Everyone goes through the blues or through a low mood that is of a passing nature. We may also feel down while trying to cope with loss or disappointments at work or at home. However, mostly in such situations after some time things get back to normal and we get back into our daily routines. These situations are not so extreme and as such don't require the services of a professional to help deal with it.

## Facts

- Depression is one of the most common mental health illnesses.
- Its prevalence among children and adolescents is estimated to be 1 per cent (Saddock, Saddock & Ruiz, 2015).
- According to the WHO, depression affects 121 million people worldwide (2011).

---

[2]It is important to note that Depression is not the same as Bipolar Disorder, in which there are cyclical periods of both high and low moods. Bipolar Disorder will be discussed at length in chapter 5.

## How can you identify depression?

By **depression**, we refer to a mood that goes well beyond just feeling the blues. Depression is a condition which involves recurrent and persistent low moods which last for at least two weeks and interfere with the affected individual's daily life and activities such as going to school and maintaining relationships with friends and family. Symptoms of depression can include the following:

- Loss of interest in activities.
- Not being able to derive pleasure from activities.
- A sense of helplessness and hopelessness about the future.
- Negative thoughts relating to the self.
- Complaints of tiredness and fatigue.
- Withdrawal from social activities.
- Interference with appetite and sleep patterns.

As individuals working closely with children it is important to understand that the signs and symptoms of depression in children and adolescents are different from those observed in adults. Since children are not competent in expressing emotions verbally, their symptoms can also involve the following:

- An increase in irritability.
- Withdrawing from activities and social interaction.
- Increase in aggression and risk-taking behaviour.
- Deterioration in academic performance.
- General appearance of sadness.
- Increase in somatic complaints like headaches and stomach aches.
- Poor self-esteem.

The general apathy, irritable mood and bleak outlook on life can be difficult and confusing for a person trying to intervene in the situation. However, it is important to treat a depressed child or teen with sensitivity while making a special effort to connect with them every day since depression is the leading cause of teenage suicide in the world, the occurrence of which, according to recent estimates, has quadrupled over the last two decades. This makes it even more imperative to effectively identify and treat the condition in the light of the fact that it is a treatable illness.

It is important to remember that depression is not due to a character weakness or something that can go away if the child 'pulls' himself together or goes through some behaviour modification. It is an illness and needs to be treated with medication and therapy. Without treatment, depression can last for weeks, months and even years, significantly impacting different spheres of an individual's life.

| Different Ways in Which Depression Can Affect a Child or Adolescent's Behaviour |
| --- |
| Social withdrawal |
| Physical complaints |
| Increase in irritability and restlessness |
| Deterioration in attention and concentration |
| Decrease in academic performance |
| Increase in risk-taking behaviour |
| Drug and alcohol use |

## What causes depression?

There is no single causative factor that can be exclusively implicated in the causation of depression. Genetic, biological and psychosocial factors all have a strong role to play in the aetiology of the illness, combining in various ways and thus leading to its precipitation.

*Biological factors:*

Biologically, the problem tends to be in the neurotransmitter levels in the brain. In depression certain neurotransmitter levels drop below normal, leading to disruption in daily life activities like sleep and appetite disturbance, low mood and loss of interest. Serotonin is one of the main neurotransmitters implicated in the causation of depressive disorders.

*Genetic factors:*

Depression also has a strong genetic component associated with it and is often seen to run in families. Research has shown that depression occurs in one in every four women in contrast to it being observed in one in every 10 men.

*Psychosocial factors:*

Many psychological and social stressors like trauma, loss of a dear one, difficulties in relationships, life-challenges, etc. can be a trigger for a depressive episode. Repeated stressful experiences tend to compromise the individual's ability to cope with the situations as they emerge, which is exacerbated if the individual does not have adequate support mechanisms in the environment.

## Why is early intervention important?

The primary reason why early intervention cannot be emphasized enough is that the early onset of the condition tends to indicate a chronic course of the illness. This would mean that we would expect a longer course of the illness as well as more episodes of depression which is associated with a poor overall prognosis. In fact, it is a well-known fact that with each episode that occurs, the chances of having more episodes only increases. This highlights the strong need to develop the right skills, coping mechanisms, support systems and getting the correct medical treatment to take care of the illness at an early stage.

Furthermore, children and adolescents who have been diagnosed with depression can develop other comorbid conditions such as anxiety, conduct disorder, alcohol and substance use which makes it increasingly challenging to treat the condition. Adequate and timely help is not always able to reach those who need it due to the existing stigma, misconceptions and myths pertaining to mental health illnesses. A major hindrance to the timely treatment of the condition is also the lack of understanding and knowledge which could facilitate timely identification.

For these reasons, **it is imperative to stop this cycle at the earliest through early identification and adequate psychiatric and psychological intervention**.

## Who is at risk?

Different children cope with difficult situations differently. Some are more resilient than others and are able to work through some of the most challenging circumstances while others may find the stresses of daily life difficult to handle, yet others may experience significant trauma that can compromise existing abilities to cope causing the onset of a depressive episode.

---

**Red Flags (Beware As These Increase Risk)**

- Parent with a history of depression or other psychiatric illness.
- Difficult and challenging family circumstances.
- History of childhood abuse—verbal, physical, or sexual.
- Low sense of self.
- Low peer-group support and other support mechanisms.
- Negative and pessimistic thinking patterns.
- Poor problem-solving and decision-making skills.
- Lack of assertiveness.

## The FSMH steps

### STEP 1: Identify the children at risk

Some behavioural signs that you need to watch out for include the following:

- Complaints of extreme fatigue even without too much physical exertion.
- Physical complaints like headaches and stomach aches.
- Always irritable or angry even without provocation.
- Expressing hopelessness or helplessness.
- Lack of concentration.
- Inability to make simple decisions.
- Talking or writing about death and suicide.
- Significant drop in grades and class performance.
- Disinterest in being with peers, preferring to be alone.
- Increase in risk-taking behaviour.
- Increase in drug and alcohol use.
- Eating too much or too little.
- Sleeping too much or too little.

It is a combination of the above mentioned aspects which would indicate the presence of depression and not the prevalence of a singular aspect.

### STEP 2: Listen non-judgementally and give reassurance

- Children or teenagers who are depressed need someone who will listen to them without judging them or offering unsolicited advice. **Active listening and engaging with the child is needed in such a scenario**. Try and empathize with the child and understand the emotional experience that he is going through. Show that you care and get your concern across to the child clearly. Many depressed children can feel expendable and unwanted, harbouring feelings of self-harm and suicide. They feel if they were to die no one would miss them. It is of great value to help such children feel like someone cares about what they are feeling and going through.

- **Do not interrogate, scold, or patronize them**. If the child is sharing his personal feelings and fears with you, respect the courage that this would take on the part of the child. Do not try to change the subject if it makes you uncomfortable. It is important for the child to share his feelings. The most effective thing that you can do at this point is to **really listen.**
- **Reflect the feelings and thoughts** that you are able to gather from the conversation you are having with the child. This conveys to the child that you are able to understand his perspective.
- **Seek clarity** where you feel confused but do not make frequent interruptions in the narrative of the child.
- **Summarize** at the end of the conversation what you have understood and reassure the child that you are available to listen and would determine a way to help the child.
- **Be accurate** in stating what you can and cannot do in case there is any discussion with the child around the same. Do not make false promises or raise the hopes and expectations of the child by stating things that you may not be able to follow through with.

## STEP 3: Determine the factors that may be responsible for the child's low mood

Various factors can be responsible for the changes that you would be noticing in the child's mood or the persistence of the low mood states. In order to work with the child it is important to have an understanding of what exactly is happening in the child's environment. To do this you need to engage in a dialogue after you have established a trusting relationship with him. In a careful manner it is important to start exploring the various aspects of his life, starting with the home, moving on to the school and finally the community.

## STEP 4: Assess the risk for suicide

Children and teens diagnosed with depression can have thoughts of attempting suicide.[3] The two most important questions that need to be asked to ascertain the risk for suicide are:

- Does the child have a current plan?
- Has there been a previous attempt?

What is important to remember is that suicide is not a sudden occurrence. It does not happen without any warning but is usually a well-thought-out decision. As a responsible adult it is very important to be aware of the cues and warning signs that precede a suicide attempt.

If you feel that a particular child or teenager is at risk, you can check the risk by direct questioning. Once you are able to engage the child in a conversation about his feelings in an honest and trusting manner, you can help the child in coping with the situation by taking a solution-oriented approach and calling upon the existing support mechanisms.

### Inform the caregiver

Having ascertained that a child or teenager is clinically depressed, it is important to talk to the caregivers and to direct them towards the right specialist to seek treatment. Providing parents

---

[3]The topics of Suicide and Self-Harm are discussed in more detail in chapter 20.

or guardians with the required information about the illness and the need for early intervention is a must as this is the only method of ensuring the right kind of help is provided to the child. Directing the parents or the guardian to the right expert forms an integral part of the treatment process.

## STEP 5: Encourage help-seeking and provide information

You can help the depressed child/teenager or their parents feel optimistic and in control of the situation by doing some basic things.

- Provide the reassurance that the symptoms being experienced are a diagnosable and treatable illness.
- It is not a character weakness or a fault.
- Being depressed is not being lazy or dependent on willpower.
- Depression can be adequately treated through psychiatric medications and counselling.

### Busting Myths Related to Depression

**Children cannot experience depression**
Depression is a mood disorder that can develop in any age group, ethnic group, economic group and gender. It impacts the individual's overall functioning and is experienced as a distressing and debilitating condition.

**Depression is just an excuse for poor behaviour**
Depression can be devastating and have a lasting effect on the child's social, emotional and cognitive development. This may result in the child behaving in ways that are inappropriate or inefficient. However, children do not have much control over their behaviour. In fact, these children who experience a change in their behaviour due to depression may feel extremely embarrassed or ashamed around others.

> **Depression is a phase that children will outgrow**
> Clinical depression is not a phase or a normal stage of development, nor something kids can shrug off. This is not just a passing bad mood. Waiting for the 'phase' to end curtails crucial early intervention, thereby resulting in more widespread and pervasive outcomes.

> **Medication is the only clinical intervention for treating childhood depression**
> Although medication is highly effective and for a majority of cases, an essential part of the treatment plan, therapeutic intervention through individual counselling using various art or play-based techniques is an equally essential element of the treatment process. Psychotherapeutic intervention is primarily focused on improving functionality, building positive self-esteem, relieving personal distress and enhancing social support.

Depression and suicidal ideation require adequate medical and psychological intervention. Professional help is irreplaceable and depression often requires medication provided by a psychiatrist.

## STEP 6: Build resilience post the intervention

What happens after the child receives treatment is as important as the treatment in itself for any kind of mental health illness. In order to effectively rehabilitate the child, it is important to make his re-integration into society as smooth as possible. Some things that you should keep in mind are:

- **Do not overtly treat the child any different from the others**, remember that other children will also take their cue from you on how to interact and behave with the child.
- **Educate the children about the illness, its signs, symptoms and effects**. Increase their awareness about the illness and the warning signs associated with feeling depressed and having thoughts of self-harm. Try to reduce

the stigma by equating mental health illnesses to physical illnesses.
- **Express hope and optimism** that the child will soon be able to perform in the same way that he previously did, and give frequent encouragement and positive strokes.
- **Encourage free expression** and help the child find a safe outlet to vent his thoughts and feelings—whether this is in the form of writing, painting, drama, or role-play.
- **Work on helping the child build good relationships** with friends and family.
- **Help the child build more effective coping mechanisms** by working on problem-solving through various brainstorming exercises and making them see solutions in problems where they do not see any.
- **Do not get discouraged if the child does not respond appreciatively to your efforts**. Hopelessness and emotional disturbance is part of the illness and usually dissipates with time if proper treatment is being provided.
- **Maintain contact with the parents and if possible with the mental health professional** to ensure that regular and consistent follow-ups are being done with regard to the illness.

Vigilance to the early signs indicating the onset or presence of depression and adherence to the steps enlisted can ensure that the child you work with receives the required intervention for his psychological health and well-being.

# 5
# BIPOLAR AND RELATED DISORDERS

**B**ipolar and related disorders essentially fall under the umbrella of mood disorders. They include disorders that share features of mood fluctuations, shifting from mania to depression, and other associated cognitive and psychomotor symptoms, and also behavioural symptoms (DSM-5, 2014). These primarily include Bipolar-I disorder, Bipolar-II disorder and Cyclothymic disorder. Other disorders such as substance/medication-induced bipolar and related disorder, bipolar and related disorder due to another medical condition, other specified bipolar and related disorder, and unspecified bipolar and related disorder are also classified under this category.

Earlier referred to as manic-depressive illness, bipolar disorders are episodic in nature in which the individual has 'episodes' of mania and/or depression. These episodes manifest as unusual shifts in mood, energy and activity levels. These fluctuations can make it hard to carry out day-to-day tasks, such as going to school or spending time with friends. Symptoms of bipolar disorder can be severe. They are different from the normal ups and downs that everyone goes through from time to time and can result in damaged relationships, poor school performance, and even suicide.

Though earlier considered rare, research suggests that the

incidence of bipolar disorders in childhood and adolescence may be equal to that seen in adults, that is, approximately 1 per cent (Lewinsohn, Klein & Seeley, 1995) of the young population. Although symptoms usually develop in the late teens or adulthood, some individuals may start showing symptoms during childhood. When the onset of bipolar disorder happens during childhood it may be more severe than in adults. Young people with bipolar disorder may show symptoms more often and switch moods more frequently than the adults who are suffering from the illness.

**Facts**

- Lifetime prevalence of Bipolar-I is 0.6 per cent, Bipolar-II is 0.4 per cent, and Bipolar spectrum (BPS) is 2.4 per cent (Merikangas, Jin, He, Kessler, Lee, Sampson, Viana et al, 2011).
- Symptom severity is greater for depressive than manic episodes (Merikangas, Jin, He, Kessler, Lee, Sampson, Viana et al, 2011).
- Three-quarters of those with BPS meet criteria for at least one other disorder, with anxiety disorders, particularly panic attacks, being the most common comorbid condition (Merikangas, Jin, He, Kessler, Lee, Sampson, Viana et al, 2011).
- Less than half of those with lifetime BPS receive mental health treatment, particularly in low-income countries where only 25 per cent of them come in contact with the mental healthcare system. (Merikangas, Jin, He, Kessler, Lee, Sampson, Viana et al, 2011).
- At least half of all cases start before the age of 25 (FDA, 2011).
- Bipolar disorder tends to run in families. Children with a parent or a sibling who has bipolar disorder are up to

six times more likely to develop the illness, compared to children who do not have a family history of bipolar disorder (Nurnberger & Foroud, 2002).
- Bipolar disorders have a high impact on daily life, with the illness usually lasting a lifetime. If left untreated, the symptoms usually get worse. However, when individuals seek treatment, and follow with a strong lifestyle that includes self-management and a good treatment plan, many people live well with the condition.

## Signs and symptoms of bipolar disorders

The individual with bipolar disorder may experience a specific and distinct manic or depressive episode, or may also have a mixed episode. There usually is a period of normal mood state between episodes, which is referred to as euthymic, wherein there is no significant or extreme mood state existing. Bipolar disorders are diagnosed when there is more than one episode of mania and/or depression. Depending on the severity, intensity, frequency of mood and other symptoms, bipolar disorders are further classified into Bipolar-I, Bipolar-II or Cyclothymic disorder.

Signs and symptoms of specific disorders are discussed below. However, before further discussion of specific disorders, it is important to understand what a distinct manic and depressive episode entails.

## Manic episode

A child having a manic episode may be overly joyful to a degree which is unusual for him. He may be extremely irritable, and have anger outbursts. He may sleep less, but not feel tired. The child may have racing thoughts and may talk a lot, really fast. He may have difficulty in paying attention and may change topics all of a sudden while talking. The child may in general engage in more activities. The behaviour may be motivated by pleasure-seeking and a risk-taking tendency. The child may also have an inflated sense of self-esteem or grandiosity. These symptoms must last for a period of one week to be considered as a manic episode.

## Hypomanic episode

The above mentioned symptoms in the manic episode, when present in a less severe or intense manner, less frequently, and lasting for less than a week, but more than four days, are classified as a hypomanic episode. The impairment in functioning is also less than as seen in a manic episode.

## Depressive episode

Depressive episode includes mood and behavioural symptoms, which are usually the opposite of a manic episode. A child or teen having a depressive episode tends to feel sad or has a low mood which lasts for at least two weeks at a stretch. He may lose interest in activities which he once enjoyed. They may report feelings of guilt, helplessness, hopelessness and worthlessness. The child may often complain of pains and aches, eat more than or less than usual, sleep more than or less than usual, feel tired often, and also experience thoughts of death and suicide. He may prefer being alone and not want to interact much with others.

### *Bipolar-I*

For a diagnosis of Bipolar-I, the individual must meet the criteria of manic episode, which may occur once or more than once. The manic episode may have been preceded by and may be followed by hypomanic or major depressive episodes.

### *Bipolar-II*

For a diagnosis of Bipolar-II, the individual must meet the criteria of at least one current or past hypomanic episode, and at least one depressive episode. Also, there should be no history of a manic episode.

### Cyclothymic disorder

For a diagnosis of Cyclothymic disorder, during a two-year period (one year in children and adolescents), there should have been numerous periods of *hypomanic symptoms* that do not meet criteria of a hypomanic episode, and periods of depressive symptoms that do not meet criteria of a depressive episode. The symptoms should be present more often than not during the two-year period. And during the same period, criteria for manic, hypomanic, or major depressive episode should not have been met.

## How can you identify bipolar disorders?

As front-line professionals dealing with mental health issues, it is important to understand that bipolar disorders are more complicated than the usual mood fluctuations or mood swings that everyone experiences as a response to positive or negative situations and life experiences. Mood swings or mood fluctuations become pathological, when they are associated with drastic behavioural changes, and the intensity, severity and frequency is not realistically related to the cause of it. Bipolar disorders not only consist of mood changes or extreme mood states, but also influence regular everyday behaviour such as the ability to pay attention and concentrate, sleep and appetite, and interpersonal relationships.

It can be difficult to identify bipolar disorder, as most of us experience mood fluctuations at some point. It is important to assess the intensity and severity of the experience, and how dysfunctional the child or adolescent is becoming in accomplishing the tasks of his everyday life.

| **Warning Signs of Bipolar Disorder** |
|---|
| • An expansive or irritable mood. |
| • Extreme sadness or lack of interest in playing. |
| • Rapidly changing moods lasting a few hours to a few days. |
| • Excessive involvement in multiple projects and activities. |
| • Impaired judgement, impulsivity, racing thoughts and the pressure to keep talking. |
| • Increased or decreased sleep. |
| • Increased or decreased appetite. |
| • Indulging in risky behaviour such as excessive spending, sexual promiscuity, or gambling. |
| • Reduced interest in activities. |
| • Tantrums or defiance. |
| • Impaired school performance. |

Bipolar disorders, particularly in the depressive phase or a hypomanic episode, may remain undiagnosed and, hence, untreated. Individuals who are suffering, as well as their family members may consider it a mood fluctuation or a behavioural phase. Particularly in developing and low-income countries, people may not seek treatment until the symptoms become severe. When there is a shift from one episode to another (such as depressive to manic episode), people may mistake it for improvement and, hence, may not seek appropriate intervention.

### What causes bipolar disorders?

Multiple theories and contributing factors have been suggested for the development of bipolar disorders. An interaction between genetic, biological, psychosocial as well as cultural factors is believed to be the cause behind the illness.

*Biological factors:*

A disturbance in the neurotransmitter levels—particularly norepinephrine and serotonin has been implicated in the causation. Fluctuation in dopamine activity (decreased in depression, and increased in mania) has also been seen to play a role in the pathophysiology of bipolar disorders. Disturbance in hormonal regulation, alterations in sleep neurophysiology, and immunological disturbances also contribute to the development of the illness.

*Genetic factors:*

The tendency to develop a bipolar disorder is also found to run in families. Family data indicate that if one parent suffers from mood disorder, a child will have a risk of between 10 to 25 per cent to develop a mood disorder. If both parents suffer, then the risk roughly doubles. However, data from twin studies suggests that genes explain only 50–70 per cent of aetiology.

*Psychological factors:*

Psychodynamic and psychosocial factors also explain the individual episodes in bipolar disorder. In terms of psychosocial factors, it is regarded that negative life events and environmental stress may result in depressive symptomatology.

## Why is early intervention important?

Considering the high level of impairment, chronicity, risk of significant negative consequences due to risky behaviour, distress and dysfunction caused by bipolar disorders—its earliest possible identification and intervention is necessary, as treatment is most effective if started in the early stages of the disorder. The longer abnormal mood states persist, the more difficult it is to overcome the disorder. Furthermore, bipolar disorders are highly comorbid with suicidal tendency.

For these reasons, **it is imperative to prevent such adverse outcomes through ensuring identification at the earliest and provision of adequate and timely psychiatric and psychological intervention.**

## Who is at risk?

Regardless of age, gender, nationality, or culture, any person can be affected by bipolar disorder. Furthermore, the severity is seen to be more when the onset is in childhood. Different individuals have different temperaments, different coping strategies and mechanisms, and deal with stressful situations in different ways. However, certain aspects contribute to a higher risk of developing bipolar disorders.

| Red Flags (Beware As These Increase Risk) |
|---|
| • Parent with a history of bipolar (or depressive) disorder.<br>• Negative life experiences.<br>• Poor coping mechanisms and low coping resources.<br>• Difficult and challenging family circumstances.<br>• High sensitivity to changes in internal and external environment.<br>• Less adaptability to change. |

## The FSMH steps

### STEP 1: Identify the children at risk

Some behavioural signs that you need to watch out for as adults working with children include:

- Irritable or expansive mood.
- Withdrawn behaviour.
- Lack of attention and concentration.

- Increased activity, doing a lot of things at once.
- Indulging in risky behaviour.
- Over-spending and overdoing things.
- Talking very fast, shifting topics frequently.
- Variety of physical complaints like palpitations and increased heartbeat.

## STEP 2: Begin a non-confrontational conversation

- **Don't hesitate to begin the conversation.** As a front-line professional who has identified a child at risk, you shouldn't hesitate in approaching them to talk about your observation and concerns. People who are experiencing such mood states, particularly during a manic episode, tend to underrate their problems, or may not feel that there is a problem, as they feel happy and, hence, don't seek treatment. As the adult in the situation, explaining to them the problem, the need for treatment and involving the family or significant others in the process can help ensure they do not ignore it and feel comfortable discussing with you.
- **Be non-confrontational.** The few people, who might have noticed their extreme mood states, might feel afraid of expressing their concerns in fear of aggressive reactions. Once you identify such behaviour, approach the child and express your observation in a non-confrontational way. Those who are suffering may be feeling weak or blaming themselves for not being 'strong enough', so even a suggestion of seeking help may feel as an attack. Be non-confrontational in your approach and make them feel accepted, while talking about their problems in terms of a disorder which can be treated. Active listening and engaging with the child is needed, to be able to express your concerns and demonstrate your support and availability to them clearly in such a scenario. Avoid being critical, as it could make them defensive as

well as defiant.
- **Be reassuring.** Most children would be anxious and insecure, and they need someone to be able to listen to them, empathize and provide reassurance. Instead, focus on the possibility of seeking help, to overcome the symptoms, and work towards a more functional lifestyle.

## STEP 3: Encourage help-seeking and provide information for the same

You can help the child and his parent/caregiver feel optimistic and in control of the situation by doing some basic things:

- Provide the reassurance that their experience is a diagnosable and treatable illness.
- Convey that recovery from a bipolar disorder is possible.
- Reassure them that bipolar disorders can be treated through adequate psychiatric and psychological interventions.

Bipolar disorders require adequate medical and psychological intervention. Effective treatment must address both the physical as well as the psychological needs of the person, and hence the role of professional help is irreplaceable. It is important to help the individual identify their triggers and to be able to determine when they are struggling which would mean developing a better understanding of the illness and what suggests the presence of an episode. Building this understanding is a crucial element of any psychological intervention.

## STEP 4: Talk to parents/caregivers

There are two scenarios in which talking to a parent or caregiver is critical. These include:

- When the child cannot understand the problem and the parents' help may be required to ensure help reaches the

child either because of the age or developmental level or because of the severity of the illness which would prevent him from being able to understand what is being communicated.
- When there is insufficient understanding on the part of the parents/caregivers which prevents the seeking or sustaining of treatment, thus, interfering with the child's recovery process.

It is going to be vital for you to psychoeducate parents and caregivers to clear the commonly held myths and beliefs related to bipolar disorders, providing them with complete information, while reassuring them about the possible courses of treatment available.

| Busting Myths Related to Bipolar Disorders |
|---|
| **Excessive happiness or unrealistic euphoria is a symptom**<br>It is important to remember that feeling happy and confident will not be considered a problem usually. Thus, explaining to the parents/caregiver the subtle differences while also highlighting the need for presence of multiple symptoms over a certain duration will help them understand and know when there is an illness. |
| **Mood swings are normal but extreme mood states may be a problem**<br>The difference between mood swings which everyone experiences and mood states in a bipolar disorder is in intensity, severity and frequency. Help them understand the shift in mood from one pole to another and the other associated symptoms, whose presence is critical in diagnosing the condition. |
| **Recovery from bipolar disorders is not possible**<br>Even though many with the diagnosis of bipolar disorder need to take treatment for a very long time, often lifelong, but with early identification and adequate and timely intervention, children with bipolar disorder can be treated and helped to lead a happier and healthier life. |

## STEP 5: Build resilience post the intervention

What happens after the individual receives treatment is as important as the treatment in itself in any kind of mental health illness. With a disorder like bipolar, it becomes all the more crucial that efforts be expended to formulate ways in which the child can be engaged with more activities and people in a bid to rehabilitate and help the child come out of the difficult episode. Some things that you should keep in mind are:

- **Express hope and optimism** to motivate the individual towards resuming a healthy lifestyle, and encourage his efforts towards the same.
- **Work on helping the person build healthy relationships** with friends and family.
- **Work with others within the child's immediate vicinity and community to understand bipolar disorder** and its treatment to effectively bust any myths related to the illness.
- **Help the child explore his talents to boost his self-confidence** and to shift his attention from things which can go wrong to things which can and do go right.
- **Help the child work towards being more cognizant of his mood states and fluctuations** which may happen and develop effective ways of being able to work on the same.
- Reinforce to the child and the family that **fear of a recurrence should not stop the child from leading his life** and that greater vigilance would suffice in ensuring that a problem can be tackled early if it arises.
- **Help the child build more effective coping mechanisms by working on problem-solving** through various brain storming exercises and make him see solutions to problems where he does not see any.
- **Encourage the child and the family to stay connected with the child's care providers** to actively work towards

maintaining the child's moods and preventing the recurrence of an episode.
- **Maintain contact with the mental health professional** to ensure that regular and consistent follow-ups are being done with regard to the illness.

Bipolar disorder can be especially debilitating, requiring the urgent attention of a professional. Awareness of how the illness manifests is instrumental in mediating its progression and impact on the lives of children.

# 6
# ANXIETY DISORDERS

It is natural for children and adolescents to feel nervous, worried or restless when faced with an unfamiliar or difficult situation. In fact, feeling anxious is one of the most common emotional states experienced across various situations in our daily lives and one that also has protective aspects associated with it. When we talk of **anxiety**, we mean a state of apprehension or unease arising out of anticipation of danger, which can be experienced in both physical as well as psychological forms. Anxiety is different from fear, as fear is an apprehension in response to external danger while in anxiety the danger is largely unknown. It is a biological mechanism of preparing our body to deal with stressful situations. It occurs in a variety of situations, such as before appearing for an exam, being away from home and family, before a significant life event, and also in situations which are unknown and non-specific.

Each child differs in his ability to cope with stressors, with some children being more resilient and being able to face challenging circumstances, as compared to others who might be easily stressed or worried. This anxiety becomes a matter of concern when the child or adolescent finds it difficult to deal with or control his anxiety, thus interfering with his functioning in academic and interpersonal aspects of life.

**Anxiety disorders** refer to those experiences, which exceed developmentally appropriate expectations, persist beyond developmentally appropriate periods, and are associated with related behavioural disturbances that typically continue for six months or more. These include generalized anxiety disorder, specific phobia, social anxiety disorder, panic disorder (and panic attacks), agoraphobia, separation anxiety disorder and selective mutism.[4]

## Facts

- A national survey of adolescent mental health by National Institute of Mental Health in 2014 reported that about 8 per cent of teens aged 13–18 years have an anxiety disorder, with symptoms commonly emerging around age of 6.
- One-year prevalence of anxiety disorders is 12.6 per cent (NIMH, 1998).
- Anxiety disorders occur more frequently in females than males, approximately in a ratio of 2:1 (APA, 2013).
- High comorbidity between anxiety and depressive disorders has been observed—30 per cent (coexisting) and 60 per cent (lifetime) (Overbeeck, Vermetten & Griez, 2001).

## Signs and symptoms of anxiety disorders

The experience of anxiety is a physiological process which begins when the child or adolescent perceives a situation to be potentially dangerous; the brain sends a message to the autonomic nervous system, thereby activating a 'fight or flight' response. The symptoms of anxiety have physical, psychological as well as behavioural manifestations.

---

[4]The topics of Separation Anxiety and Selective Mutism are discussed in detail in chapters 7 and 8, respectively.

| Signs and Symptoms of Anxiety | | |
|---|---|---|
| Physical | Psychological | Behavioural |
| Breathlessness | Lack of attention and concentration | Fatigue |
| Sweating | | Restlessness |
| Heart pounding | Deficits in memory | Irritability |
| Trembling | Feeling of losing control | Disturbed sleep |
| Involuntary urination | | Avoidance of specific anxiety-evoking situations |
| Numbness or tingling sensations | Fear of going crazy/dying | |
| | Ruminations and constant worrying | Excessive reassurance seeking |
| Dizziness | Low self-esteem | Disturbed interpersonal relations |
| Indigestion | All-or-none thinking[5] | |
| Headache | | |
| Dryness of mouth | | |
| Nausea and vomiting | | |

Besides the general manifestations of anxiety, the features of some specific anxiety disorders in children and adolescents are as follows:

*Specific phobia:*

- Persistent fear of a specific object or situation. For example, a dog, heights, or blood.
- The fear is unreasonable and out of proportion to the actual danger.
- The child gets anxious whenever confronting or anticipating the object or situation.
- The child makes efforts to avoid the feared object or situation.

---

[5] All-or-none thinking is a cognitive error in which the person views everything in extremes or black and white, while ignoring the rest.

*Social anxiety disorder (social phobia):*

- Persistent fear of a social or performance situation in the presence of unfamiliar people.
- The child fears being scrutinized or negatively evaluated.
- The child gets anxious whenever confronting or anticipating the situation.
- The child makes efforts to avoid the situation.

*Panic disorder:*

- Repeated and unexpected **panic attacks**.
   - A panic attack is a sudden and intense fear or discomfort which rises to a peak within minutes, with physical manifestations of anxiety including a pounding heart, sweating, trembling of hands, feeling of being choked, and psychological symptoms including fear of losing control, going crazy, or dying.
- The child is worried about having a panic attack and its consequences.
- The child's behaviour changes in effort to avoid situations or circumstances where he fears the onset of a panic attack.

*Agoraphobia:*

- The child experiences anxiety about being in places from which escape might be difficult or in which help may not be available. For example, fear of using public transport, being in enclosed or open spaces, standing in a queue or crowd.
- The child avoids these situations fearing that something terrible might happen to him.

*Generalized anxiety disorder:*

- The child has excessive anxiety and worries about a number of events.
- The child is not able to control his worry.
- The worry is accompanied by situations of restlessness,

irritability, fatigue, difficulty concentrating or the mind going blank, sleep disturbance, or muscle tension.

## How can you identify anxiety disorders?

You may have witnessed many children or adolescents getting nervous, anxious, or very worried in situations like examinations or in a social situation when in front of many people. It is crucial to be able to determine when this anxiety is exceeding in intensity and is persisting beyond the developmentally normative expectations and impacting the overall functioning of the child in a way that it is impeding his ability to take care of his daily routines, chores and tasks expected of him.

It is important to understand that the signs and symptoms of anxiety in children and adolescents can be different from those observed in adults. Since children are not always able to express emotions verbally with ease, their symptoms can frequently manifest in their behaviour in a variety of ways. In fact, while some anxious children would become evasive and avoidant, others might react with an overwhelming need to break out of an uncomfortable situation in the form of temper tantrums, anger, or aggression. As someone working closely with children it is vital to be able to identify these warning signs of anxiety which can be easily inferred by observing their behaviour.

| Warning Signs of Anxiety Disorder |
| --- |
| • Restlessness and nervousness |
| • Excessive worrying |
| • Change in social interactions or sudden clinging behaviour |
| • Hyper-vigilance and over-cautiousness |
| • Frequent physical complaints |
| • Not engaging in routine activities unless the parent is available |
| • Avoiding specific situations because of worry or fear |

| |
|---|
| • Disturbances in sleep patterns |
| • Poor concentration |
| • Being irritable |

## What causes anxiety disorders?

The following biological, genetic and psychosocial factors have been implicated in the precipitation of the various anxiety disorders.

*Biological factors:*

Anxiety disorders involve a disruption in the regulation of neurotransmitters. Studies have shown that alteration in the levels of these neurotransmitters may lead to clinical anxiety.

*Genetic factors:*

The tendency to develop an anxiety disorder is also found to run in families. While no specific gene has been implicated in their development, research suggests that an individual with a family member having an anxiety disorder is more susceptible to develop the same. Such individuals are likely to inherit temperamental traits such as shyness, hyperactive autonomic nervous systems, or behavioural inhibition from their anxious family members, thereby leading to a predisposition to develop the condition.

*Psychosocial factors:*

Psychological and social stressors like trauma, loss of a dear one, difficulties in relationships, pressure relating to academics, adverse changes in the environment and other life-challenges can be a trigger for symptoms of anxiety. Repeated stressful experiences tend to compromise the individual's ability to cope with situations as they emerge, which is exacerbated if the individual does not have adequate support mechanisms in the environment. Further, chronic or ongoing stressful events also play a major role in maintaining the symptoms once the condition has been triggered.

## Why is early intervention important?

Considering the amount of distress caused by anxiety disorders, and their adverse impact on the child or adolescent's academic, social, as well as personal functioning, the earliest possible identification and intervention is of undeniable importance. Treatment is most effective if started in the early stages of the disorder, before maladaptive behaviour patterns take hold. The longer abnormal anxiety behaviour persists, the more difficult it is to overcome the disorder. Furthermore, anxiety disorders are highly comorbid with depressive disorders and it can increase the tendency to avoid and escape from important situations where anxiety may present itself, like at school or with friends or outside the home. Hence, it is important that timely intervention is provided, to prevent these negative consequences.

## Who is at risk?

Each child is different and unique, varying in abilities to deal with anxiety-provoking situations using different coping strategies and mechanisms. However, some children are often at a greater risk of developing difficulties in coping, increasing their chances of experiencing anxiety related problems.

| Red Flags (Beware As These Increase Risk) |
|---|
| • Parent with a history of anxiety disorder or any other psychiatric illness.<br>• Low sense of self, poor self-esteem, or self-confidence.<br>• Multiple disappointments in situations involving evaluation.<br>• Introverted or shy temperament, preventing sharing and discussing of problems. |

- History of substance use.
- Anxious, insecure, or perfectionist disposition.
- Difficult and challenging family circumstances.
- Low peer group and family support and other support mechanisms.

**The FSMH steps**

**STEP 1: Identify the children at risk**

As we discussed, anxiety is a commonly expected natural response in many situations and it can serve numerous protective functions as well, by making one aware of the threats or challenges that a situation posits. However, this normal amount of anxiety can be a significant problem if it exceeds what is normally expected given the situation, the age of the child and his expected coping resources. It is, thus, important for you to be able to identify the children whose behaviour is diverging from reasonable and developmentally appropriate expectations. Besides the warning signs mentioned above, some common examples of behaviour that signal an anxiety disorder include:

- Being startled easily.
- Avoiding specific situations repeatedly.
- Feeling anxious and apprehensive generally.
- Needing the constant support of parents or other adults.
- Frequent physical complaints like headaches and stomach aches.
- Appearing irritable or angry even without provocation.
- Difficulty in concentrating.
- Inability to take simple decisions.
- Drop in grades and class performance.
- Drug and alcohol use.
- Eating too much or too little.

- Sleeping too much or too little.
- Becoming over-cautious.
- Constantly seeking reassurance.

## STEP 2: Talk to the child

- **Build trust and rapport with the child.** It is common to come across anxious children who are likely to be defensive, may not communicate and share and, therefore, it is very important for you to be able to gain the child's trust. Being able to talk to someone about their inner thoughts and feelings itself can be an anxiety-provoking situation for such children, so the child would naturally avoid talking about his problems. Therefore, it is important for the child to develop a rapport and a trusting relationship with you.
- **Listen to the child.** Children or teenagers who are anxious need someone who will listen to them without judging them or offering unsolicited advice. Active listening and engaging with the child is needed to be able to express your concerns and demonstrate your support and availability. Anxious children might ask you the same questions repeatedly, and it is important for you to be patient, while helping to allay their doubts and put their minds at ease.
- **Empathize with the child by reflecting accurately.** While talking to the child, it is helpful to reflect his thoughts and feelings that you are able to gather from the conversation. This would not only convey to the child that you are able to understand his perspective, but also help in calming the current level of anxiety.
- **Be non-confrontational.** Once you identify such behaviour, it is important to approach the child showing your genuine concern and at the same time acknowledging their problems. Anxious children might have had difficult experiences with the few people who may have noticed their anxiety, and they

are likely to feel weak or blame themselves for not being 'strong enough' to cope with their stresses effectively. Being non-confrontational in your approach would make them feel accepted and less fearful of having an interaction with you.
- **Provide reassurance.** Anxious children usually harbour feelings of insecurity and fear. Therefore, as the adult who is engaging with the child, it is important for you to provide reassurance and comfort. It is helpful to talk about their problems in terms of a diagnosable disorder which has causes beyond their personal control, being medical in nature and which can be treated effectively using both medications and counselling.

## STEP 3: Determine the factors that may be responsible for the child's anxiety

Anxiety can occur on account of multiple factors which in combination with each other can give rise to a complicated clinical picture as well. It is easy to feel that a child's behaviour or his lack of performance may be a reflection of laziness or disinterest; however, anxiety too could be playing a significant role in the development of the problem. In such a scenario, before discussing with the parents it is essential to elicit from the child what factors other than biological factors, that is, neurotransmitters or genetics, may be involved in the development or maintenance of the anxiety. It is important to start exploring the various aspects of the child's life in a careful manner, starting with the home, moving on to the school, and finally the community—laying emphasis on the child's perspective on every situation.

## STEP 4: Use art to develop an understanding

Children diagnosed with anxiety disorders show deficits in their ability to communicate their emotions freely to others around them. Using creative art-based methodologies (dance, music, writing and art) is an effective way due to its indirect and non-threatening approach to emotional expression and regulation. The goal of using art with children diagnosed with anxiety disorders in not only to put them at ease and focus their thoughts and energy on a calming outlet, but to also help foster their self-esteem, interpersonal relationships and communication with others.

When children are invested in expressing their feelings in a creative way, they are able to distract themselves from negative and anxiety-provoking thoughts. Creative art-based work helps the individual to be involved and engaged with the creative process without any interference. The key to an effective art-based session is to identify what material the child is drawn to or stimulated by—crayons and paper, music and instruments, movement and dance, craft and clay, journaling and poetry. This helps to utilize the art form closest to the child to both build trust and create activities that foster expression, communication and primarily relaxation, while eventually building coping abilities.

## STEP 5: Talk to parents/caregivers

It would be essential for you to inform the parents or caregivers about the signs you have been observing, not only helping them understand how difficult and challenging it is for the child to experience these feelings, but also to psychoeducate them to clear the common myths related to anxiety disorders and mental health problems. The aim is to provide them with complete information, while reassuring them about the possible courses of treatment available.

| |
|---|
| **Busting Myths Related to Anxiety Disorder** |
| **Excessive anxiety is just overreacting or being shy and introverted** <br> It is important to remember that anxiety disorder is not merely overreacting to a stressful situation. Rather, anxiety disorders require pharmacological and psychological intervention to help the child or adolescent overcome the distress caused by it. |
| **Anxiety disorders are a personality trait which can't be changed** <br> Anxiety disorders are a serious illness with underlying physical and psychological aspects. Such anxious children and adolescents need appropriate intervention to help them develop better coping mechanisms and overcome their anxiety. |
| **Recovery from anxiety disorders is not possible** <br> With early identification and adequate and timely intervention, an individual with an anxiety disorder can be treated and helped to lead a happier and healthier life. |

## STEP 6: Encourage help-seeking and provide information

- After talking to the child and his parents/caregivers, it is also necessary to **show them the path forward,** in terms of management of the condition as well as the things that they need to keep in mind while dealing with the condition themselves.
- **Help the child or the parents feel optimistic and in control of the situation** by providing them the reassurance that anxiety disorders are treatable.
- It is important for you to **help the parents as well as the child to realize that effective treatment for anxiety disorders must address both the physical as well as the psychological needs,** and hence the role of professional

help is irreplaceable.
- **Help the parents understand that their child should not be scolded, mocked, or forced to perform or engage in activities that he is anxious or apprehensive about.** Instead it is important to discuss and provide support and guidance so that the child can feel comfortable and may be able to still engage in activities, previously feared, due to the support from the family.

## STEP 7: Build resilience post the intervention

What happens after the child receives treatment is as important as the treatment itself. In order to take care of the impact the problem has on the child and his life, focus needs to be directed at his reintegration into his everyday life and routine. Some things that you should keep in mind and instil in others who closely interact with the child are:

- **A child who has a tendency to get anxious needs to be encouraged to find a safe outlet to vent his thoughts and feelings**—whether this is in the form of writing, painting, drama, or role-play.
- **Efforts should be made to build secure attachments with the child,** and to build good relationships with friends and family.
- **Express hope and optimism to motivate the child** towards resuming a healthy lifestyle, and encourage his efforts towards the same.
- **Provide more outlets and avenues for experiencing a sense of mastery** which would help build the child's sense of self and self-esteem.
- **Encourage the child to take on responsibilities** that would enable him to experience a sense of heightened self-worth, while also aiding him in identifying his strengths and giving a sense of positivity.

- **Help the child build more effective coping mechanisms** by working on problem-solving and encouraging discussions in both individual and group settings.
- **It is important to educate other children**, to increase their awareness about such problems and discourage their mocking behaviour which may affect how the child views himself.
- **Continue to expose the child to previously feared situations, people and stimuli gradually,** helping the child realize that his anxiety did not have any rational or logical basis.
- **Reiterate on a regular basis the biological part of anxiety disorders** and the role that avoidance plays in increasing fear.
- Finally, it is absolutely necessary for you to **maintain contact with the parents/guardian and if possible with the mental health professional** to ensure that regular and consistent follow-ups are being done post-intervention and that there is no returning to previous maladaptive patterns of behaving and responding.

## STEP 8: Take a preventive approach—build life skills

A focus also needs to be on taking a preventive approach and making children resilient towards the development of problems like anxiety disorders. One of the most effective mechanisms to achieve this goal is through the utilization of life skills programs which teach children effective skills to lead a healthy life, making them resilient and in a better position to face difficulties and challenges, thus, enhancing their coping abilities. Whether these are done through large group interactions or through the medium of small workshops and skill-based sessions, these go a long way in ensuring that a child is more insulated from developing a mental health problem.

# 7

# SEPARATION ANXIETY

It is common for young children to cry, throw temper tantrums, not want to be separated from the people they are attached to—all of which happens as part of their normal mental growth and development. Such tendencies are typically outgrown by most children as they advance through the developmental cycle. However, some children can be seen to be extremely anxious, distressed even when only anticipating a separation from their parents/caregivers and would cry a lot and not be soothed easily in such a situation.

A child is diagnosed with **separation anxiety disorder** when he has an excessive fear concerning separation from home or from those to whom he is attached. This anxiety is inappropriate for the child's developmental age, and persists for at least four weeks. Moreover, the child would usually fear as well as avoid any anticipated separation, would worry about the well-being of the attached figures, consequently leading to disruption in his daily activities.

## Facts

- The rate of separation anxiety disorder is estimated to be about 4 per cent in children and young adolescents (Saddock, Saddock & Ruiz, 2015).

- Onset of separation anxiety disorder may be as early as preschool age and may occur at any time during childhood and more rarely in adolescence (APA, 2013).

## How can you identify separation anxiety disorder?

A child having separation anxiety would not only get excessively distressed when separated from home or any attachment figure, but would exhibit fear even when anticipating such a separation. Such children typically worry about the well-being of these attachment figures whenever they are not around, fearing the occurrence of some harm or mishap. As a result of their intense anxiety, these children would go to any extent to avoid going to school or to be left alone at any place which would distance them from the attachment figures. It is not uncommon to hear frequent complaints of stomach aches, vomiting, or other somatic complaints in order to avoid separation. They would even need someone to be next to them at night, also frequently having nightmares during their sleep.

As the adult working with children, it is important for you to be aware of the various behavioural signs which could be a manifestation of an underlying separation anxiety in the child.

| Warning Signs of Separation Anxiety |
|---|
| • Irregular attendance |
| • Decline in academic performance |
| • Difficulty in developing and maintaining friendships |
| • Temper tantrums/defiance towards separation |
| • Frequent somatic/physical complaints |
| • Disturbed sleep/nightmares |
| • Low self esteem |
| • Difficulty in concentrating |

## What causes separation anxiety?

While separation anxiety is a universal phenomenon as a part of normal human development emerging in infants less than 1 year of age, but persistence of such an excessive fear of separation can be a result of a combination and interaction of biological, genetic and psychosocial factors.

*Biological factors:*

The role of certain neurotransmitters in the brain has been clearly implicated in the development of anxiety disorders, especially a chemical imbalance involving two specific neurotransmitters called norepinephrine and serotonin. Moreover, neuro-physiological factors like higher resting heart rates and elevated salivary cortisol levels have also been found to be related to extremely shy and inhibited children.

*Genetic factors:*

Research studies have suggested that separation anxiety may be heritable, with a higher tendency for those with members in the family already having a history of anxiety disorders.

*Psychosocial factors:*

Psychosocial factors in conjunction with a child's shy temperament may influence the degree of separation anxiety the child is likely to experience. Often frequent shifting of neighbourhood and exposure to unfamiliar situations can make the child insecure and more prone to developing separation anxiety. Many psychological and social stressors in the environment, like trauma, loss of a dear one, difficulties in relationships, or other life-challenges, could be factors contributing to anxiety. Furthermore, over-protectiveness and intrusive behaviour of parents can also increase the chances of separation anxiety in their child.

## Why is early intervention important?

The persistence of the symptoms of separation anxiety can deter the child's smooth transition into other social arenas. This can significantly impact the child's ability to adapt and adopt a new environment such as going to school or going for a class or activity. At the same time, the longer the symptoms are left untreated, the more challenging it is to overcome them and the impact they have upon other facets of the child's life such as interpersonal relationships with friends or family or on academics can be quite great. These factors make it essential that the earliest intervention be made when first symptoms of separation anxiety are observed.

## Who is at risk?

Every child would feel uncomfortable in an unfamiliar situation without parents/caregivers around. However, different children cope with difficult situations differently. Some are more resilient than others and are able to work through some of the most challenging circumstances while others may find the stressors of daily life difficult to handle. Some children are often at a greater risk of developing difficulties in coping, increasing their chances of experiencing anxiety.

| Red Flags (Beware As These Increase Risk) |
|---|
| • Parent with a history of anxiety or other psychiatric illness.<br>• Unstable family circumstances.<br>• Loss of or separation from an attachment figure.<br>• Low sense of self.<br>• Low peer-group support and other support mechanisms.<br>• Overprotective or neglectful parenting. |

## The FSMH steps

### STEP 1: Identify the children at risk

You would have come across a situation in which the child is not willing to let go of his parents, especially in the initial days when the child joins a new activity or a school or playschool. However, it is important for you to be able to identify the children whose behaviour is developmentally inappropriate and indicates towards it being a clinical problem which would require a formal intervention. Besides the warning signs mentioned above, some common examples of behaviours that signal the problem of separation anxiety include:

- Clinging to parents/caregivers.
- Crying/irritability/anger when separated from the primary attachment figure.
- Frequent excuses or physical complaints to avoid separation.
- Constantly seeking attention of the primary attachment figure.

### STEP 2: Help the parents understand the problem

It is a must that the parents understand the problem at length and are able to see that it is not something which would resolve on its own. Often parents consider these symptoms as a phase that every child goes through without realizing how agonizing and tormenting it is for the child to experience these feelings. Therefore, it is very important for them to be well-informed so that proper treatment and care can be provided to the child.

| Busting Myths Related to Separation Anxiety |
|---|
| **Separation anxiety is normal** |
| While experiences of anxiety when not in the presence of attachment figures is a normative phase of development, anxiety which exceeds the developmental stage can be a diagnosable separation anxiety disorder. |

> **Children clinging to parents should be reprimanded**
> Children who are having separation anxiety are likely to exhibit clinging behaviour towards the parents/caregivers. Such behaviour is a sign of their fear and insecurity, and reprimands would only scare the child further. Instead, the child needs to be reassured.

> **Children always outgrow separation anxiety**
> A child who is experiencing developmentally inappropriate separation anxiety would typically require adequate and timely interventions in order to overcome such fears.

## STEP 3: Rule out the presence of any other psychological or emotional problem the child may be having

It is important to remember that when separation anxiety develops, particularly at a later stage of mental growth, there could be other problems precipitating it. It has been observed that such a response can occur in case the child is experiencing any other significant emotional or psychological issue as well. These can stem from problems like abuse or bullying and it would be imperative that if you are identifying the presence of separation anxiety in the child, you must explore and ensure that any other such factors are not present which are complicating the situation and creating the need in the child to cling to the primary attachment figure in order to feel more secure.

## STEP 4: Work with the parents to understand and develop simple effective steps to tackle the problem

Helping a child with separation anxiety requires a very detailed understanding from the parents or caregivers about the child's experiences, the home environment, parenting practices, frequency of the problem behaviour and ways in which they have tried to work on this problem with the child previously. It also requires empathy from the family and all other adults who spend time with the child. It would be important to help the parents develop a strategy to tackle the problem. Some of the basic things which they can start with include the following:

- **Encourage the parents to start with small steps and leave the child with other adults** or on their own, starting with the home first. It could start with the parents moving to another room while another individual stays with the child and then building up the practice slowly.
- **Comforting the child should be encouraged** but it should be ensured that there is no excessive indulgence in comforting on the parents account.
- It is important that **once the child has been comforted the parent needs to explain to the child the need to move away** and then try it again after some time so that the child understands that each time the parent goes he/she does come back.
- **Parents should provide reassurance to the child that they come back** even if they do leave for a little while.
- **Reward systems can also be developed in order to encourage the child** to separate from the parent and control his distress.
- **Punishment should be avoided** in order to try and teach the child that it is ok to separate from the parent.

## STEP 5: Encourage help-seeking and provide information

If the situation is not getting resolved despite your efforts in collaboration with the parent or if there are other additional factors which are causing the onset and maintenance of the problem, it would be advisable to encourage the parents to seek additional counsel. Meeting with an external professional should be used to take care of other external aspects impinging upon the child's well-being besides the core issue of anxiety. After talking to the child and his parents/caregivers, it is necessary to show them the path for the future. They need to be reassured with complete and correct information, knowing whom to seek help from and being aware of the possible courses of action required. You should help the parents realize that their child should not be scolded or mocked and that he would need their patient support and guidance.

## STEP 6: Building resilience post the intervention

It is important to recognize that at the bottom of separation anxiety is plain anxiety. A child who has a tendency to get anxious needs to be encouraged to find a safe outlet to give vent to his thoughts and feelings as they arise. Anxiety related issues in young children can best be addressed by helping the child develop a sense of security in disclosing information about how he feels, while also working with him on solving the problems. At the same time, efforts should be made to help the child build strong, supportive relationships with more people rather than being restricted to a few adults in his surroundings.

# 8

# SELECTIVE MUTISM

Anxiety manifests itself in various forms. Some children tend to be shy, some avoid evaluation, some run behind their parents and other adults, and some tend to simply go absolutely quiet. Often mistaken as a variant of introversion or shyness, there are children who can have a condition which is known as **selective mutism**.

Selective mutism is an anxiety disorder found in children that involves continuous failure of the child to speak in certain social situations. The child knows the language and is able to speak otherwise, however, he becomes selectively mute only in those specific situations. For example, such a child would typically become quiet or may not speak at all during social outings or in school, being interactive at other times at home or with a select few people.

## Facts

- Selective mutism is a relatively rare disorder, with a prevalence of 0.03–1 per cent depending on the setting, for example it's more common in a hospital, school, or among a large crowd (APA, 2013).
- The onset of selective mutism is usually before the age of 5, being more likely to manifest in children than in adolescents

or adults (DSM-5, 2014).
- Although its duration often lasts for several months, but if left untreated it may sometimes persist for longer and may continue for years (APA, 2000).

## How can you identify selective mutism?

It is common to see children who are relatively shy and timid, preferring to keep to themselves. However, it is important to be aware of the signs to identify a selectively mute child so that the right kind of intervention can be provided to take care of the condition.

| Warning Signs of Selective Mutism |
|---|
| • Appears unwilling or hesitant to reply despite repeated attempts. |
| • Doesn't initiate conversations in social situations. |
| • Speaks spontaneously in other situations. |
| • Avoidant of social or performance situations. |
| • Excessively shy or clingy. |
| • Throws temper tantrums. |

## What causes selective mutism?

As is the case in other anxiety disorders, multiple theories and contributing factors have been suggested for selective mutism as well. However, no single causative factor has been fully implicated. Its aetiology involves an interaction between genetic, biological and psychosocial factors.

*Biological factors:*

The role of neurotransmitters has been clearly established in the causation of anxiety disorders. Alterations in their levels can lead to the precipitation of the condition.

*Genetic factors:*

Most anxiety disorders have a tendency to run in the family. Children with at least one parent having any anxiety disorder have higher chances of being diagnosed with selective mutism.

*Psychosocial factors:*

Besides the biological and genetic factors, many psychological and social stressors like trauma, loss of a dear one, difficulties in relationships, stress related to academics, change in environment, and other life-challenges can be a trigger for symptoms of anxiety. Moreover, over-protective, controlling or detached parenting can also increase the chances of children developing selective mutism.

**Why is early intervention important?**

The challenge with a problem like selective mutism is the possibility of the transfer to anxiety to other situations, thus generalizing to more situations than where it first emerged. At the same time, a problem like selective mutism interferes with many other significant aspects of a child's growth and development. For instance, for a child who is displaying signs of selective mutism it is possible that social interactions and relationships are being disrupted at school on account of the child's anxiety there. This makes it imperative that an early intervention be engaged in as the passage of time only strengthens the symptoms, making it difficult to dislodge them.

## Who is at risk?

In addition to the above mentioned factors, there are certain other factors that tend to increase the risk of a child developing selective mutism.

| Red Flags (Beware As These Increase Risk) |
|---|
| • Parental history of shyness, social inhibition or any anxiety disorder.<br>• Anxious or insecure disposition.<br>• Difficult and challenging family circumstances.<br>• History of childhood abuse—verbal, physical, or sexual.<br>• Low sense of self.<br>• Low peer group support and other support mechanisms.<br>• Over-protective, controlling, or detached parenting. |

## The FSMH steps

### STEP 1: Identify the children at risk

While many children have a tendency to prefer remaining silent in the presence of authority figures outside home, as an adult working with children it is important to be aware of certain behavioural signs that could indicate the child is at risk for selective mutism. In addition to the warning signs discussed previously, the following could help in identifying the children at risk:
- Discomfort in the presence of unfamiliar others.
- Persistent lack of communication despite being in an environment for a considerable period of time.
- Excessive clinging to parents.
- Few or no friends.
- Crying or displaying anger if forced to speak.
- Avoidance of social situations.

## STEP 2: Talk to parents/caregivers

As you work directly with children and their families, it would be common to face parents or caregivers who would be unaware of what selective mutism is. More often than not, it is likely to be viewed as shyness that the child is expected to outgrow in time. Therefore, after having identified that the child is displaying the characteristic signs and symptoms of selective mutism, it is important to inform the parents and caregivers and get them on board with the diagnosis so as to be able to direct them to the right specialist for treatment. It is vital for you to psychoeducate them, providing them with complete information, while reassuring them about the possible courses of treatment available.

Encourage parents to remove the pressure on the child to speak and ask them not to force the child to speak. It is essential to help the parents calm down, talk in a non-confrontational manner and give them time to accept the fact that their child may be suffering from a problem. Providing parents or guardians with the required information about the illness and the need for early intervention is a must as this is the only method of ensuring that the right kind of help is provided to the child.

> **Busting Myths Related to Selective Mutism**
>
> **A child with selective mutism will speak if pressured**
> Selective mutism is an anxiety disorder due to which the child is unable to speak in specific situations. On the contrary, being forced or pressured to speak is likely to increase the selectively mute child's anxiety. Instead, support and encouragement are more helpful.

| **Selective mutism is just being overly shy** |
|---|
| Selective mutism is much more extreme than ordinary shyness. It is a diagnosable disorder. The child's anxiety begins to interfere with academic, social and personal functioning. |
| **The child can outgrow selective mutism with age** |
| A selectively mute child would not simply 'outgrow' his anxiety. Selective mutism is an anxiety disorder that requires adequate psychiatric as well as psychological intervention to be treated. |

## STEP 3: Talk to the child

- **Don't hesitate to begin the conversation.** A child with selective mutism is unlikely to be willing to speak to you. Such a situation makes it all the more challenging to be able to initiate a conversation. Nevertheless, it is important for you to talk to the child. These children would typically have been struggling within themselves for quite some time. Therefore, you could approach the child showing your genuine concern, and at the same time demonstrating your understanding of the nature of the child's problems. It is of great value to help such children by helping them realize that someone does understand and care about what they are feeling and experiencing. You can also use alternate mediums for communicating with the child like signs or even art and play activities.
- **Build trust and rapport with the child.** Children with selective mutism are so anxious that they are likely to be wary and defensive in talking to most people. Therefore, it is very important for you to be able to gain the child's trust and confidence.
- **Shift your conversation from the problem to other aspects.** Having a conversation about their problems continuously would also be an anxiety-provoking situation for such children. Thus, once the initial contact has been

made and understanding of the problem communicated it would be important to shift the conversation to neutral topics till the child feels comfortable to broach difficult subjects himself.

- **Do not force the child to speak.** It is necessary to remember that coaxing an anxious child to speak up is only likely to increase his anxiety levels. It is probable for children with selective mutism to have faced situations in which they have been forced and prodded to speak, which would make them more rigid about not communicating with you as well. It is, thus, vital for you to show an acceptance towards the child's silence.
- **Maintain your patience in your attempts to communicate with the child.** Give the child the time he wants to take to become comfortable with you. As someone working closely with the child, you need to be calm and patient, allowing the child the time to open up with you.
- **Provide reassurance.** Selectively mute children are likely to harbour feelings of insecurity and fear. Therefore, as the adult engaging with the child, it is helpful to talk about their problems in terms of a diagnosable disorder which has causes beyond their control and, which can be treated effectively.

## STEP 4: Use creative art-based mediums to communicate with the child

A child displaying selective mutism is experiencing considerable anxiety and would find it challenging to communicate with people in social situations through the use of verbal mediums. You will see the child more often being comfortable in using signs to communicate what he needs. When a selectively mute child is provided with alternate mediums like art, play, music, and the like, they are able to put aside their anxiety and can channelize it to indicate what may be happening through these alternate methods. Besides helping you form a good rapport and to gain the child's trust, this would also facilitate the process of enhancing your understanding of the child and his experiences.

## STEP 5: Encourage help-seeking and provide information

Parents and caregivers are likely to be apprehensive about the further course of action for their child. It is important for you to help them realize that selective mutism in children requires adequate medical and psychological intervention clearly indicating that the professional help of a psychiatrist and a psychologist is irreplaceable. Both the parents as well as the child need to be reassured with complete and correct information, knowing whom to seek help from and being aware of the possible courses of action required. You should help the parents realize that their child should not be forced or mocked, and instead be given their support. It is helpful to reassure them that selective mutism is an illness like any other which can be treated, while clarifying all their doubts patiently.

## STEP 6: Build resilience post the intervention

During and post the intervention for selective mutism, it is important to make the child's experiences in his school and community as smooth as possible. Some of the things that would facilitate the process and also enhance the child's resilience include:

- **Do not overtly treat the child any different from the others,** remember that other children will also take cue from you on how to interact and behave with the child.
- **Do not push the child to perform or interact** and allow the child the space to be able to increase his communication

at his own pace.
- **Provide opportunities and options to the child to be expressive** using mediums other than verbal language. For instance, the child can be allowed to write an answer on the board instead of orally answering the same.
- **Encourage the child with positive statements** and usage of other reinforcers.
- **Encourage free expression and help the child find a safe outlet to vent his thoughts and feelings**—whether this is in the form of writing, painting, drama, or role-play.
- **Promote emphasis on establishing an active support system for the child,** helping the child build good relationships with friends and family. This can be proactively done with other children of the same age by using the buddy system or by requesting another child in the community to be friendly with the selectively mute child.
- A significant amount of help and support can be provided to children if **awareness is spread in schools, homes and in the social network**. Once parents, teachers and relatives become aware of the problem, it can be ensured that everyone interacting with the child is following the same approach to help with the child's anxiety.
- **Maintain contact with the parents and if possible with the mental health professional** to ensure that regular and consistent follow-ups are being done to take care of the problem.

The varied manifestations of anxiety in forms like selective mutism make it essential to be aware of how it can be identified and eliminated from a child's repertoire of responding to people and situations. Active engagement with the problem utilizing the diverse methodologies listed above can prove to be of a significant support.

# 9
# OBSESSIVE-COMPULSIVE DISORDER

Children can be stubborn and prefer their own fixed way of doing things. They frequently have their idiosyncratic ideas and thought processes about how things should be. Many also tend to have certain habits and preoccupations that they may follow very conscientiously. It is only when these begin to cause hindrance in their day-to-day functioning, impairing daily routines, requiring substantial periods of time for completion that it may indicate the presence of a problem, namely, **obsessive-compulsive disorder** (OCD).

The diagnosis of OCD is made only when the child or adolescent experiences repetitive, intrusive thoughts, ideas, or images. In effort to overcome the anxiety and distress that is caused by these intrusions, the child might indulge in some types of behaviour repeatedly in a bid to neutralize the thought. The preoccupation with these intrusions and/or the associated repetitive actions leads to significant disruption in the child's personal, social and occupational functioning.

### Facts

- OCD is one of the top 20 causes of illness-related disability, worldwide, for individuals between 15 and 44 years of age (WHO, 2009).

- The lifetime prevalence of OCD in India has been found to be 0.6 per cent (Khanna, Gururaj & Sriram, 2009).
- One-third of adults with OCD develop the symptoms in their childhood (NIMH, 2013).
- Studies of OCD in children and adolescents show males outnumber females in India (Reddy, Srinath, Prakash, Girimaji, Sheshadri & Khanna, 2003).
- Most common obsessions and compulsions in children are cleaning (32–87 per cent), followed by repetition, checking, and aggressive thoughts (Geller, Biederman, Jones, Shapiro, Schwartz & Park, 1998).

## Signs and symptoms of obsessive-compulsive disorder

The characteristic feature of OCD is the presence of **obsessions**, that is, repetitive, intrusive thoughts, ideas and images that produce uneasiness, apprehension, anxiety and fear or worry. Frequently associated with these obsessions are **compulsions,** which is repetitive behaviour aimed at reducing the associated tension or anxiety caused by the obsessions.

Common examples of obsessions and compulsions include the following:

### Obsessions

- Constant, irrational worry about dirt, germs, or contamination of self or belongings.
- Excessive concern with order, arrangement, or symmetry of objects.
- Excessive concern or fear about accidentally or purposefully causing harm to self or others.
- Excessively doubting self or others.

## Compulsions

- Cleaning: repeatedly washing one's hands, bathing, or cleaning household items, often for hours at a time.
- Checking: checking and re-checking several times a day that the doors are locked, the gas-stove is turned off, repeatedly revising homework, etc.
- Repeating: inability to stop repeating a name, phrase, or simple activity (such as climbing the staircase in a particular order, or retracing steps back and forth, rereading, erasing or rewriting).
- Hoarding: difficulty throwing away useless items such as old newspapers or magazines, bottle caps, or rubber bands.
- Ordering: repeatedly touching and re-arranging furniture or other objects in effort to gain symmetry and order.
- Mental rituals: endless reviewing of conversations; counting; repetitively recalling 'good' thoughts to neutralize 'bad' thoughts; or excessive praying and using special words or phrases to neutralize obsessions.

## How can you identify obsessive-compulsive disorder?

Identifying the symptoms of obsessive-compulsive disorder can be difficult, as the obsessive or compulsive behaviour is most likely to be interpreted as rigidity and defiance on the part of the child. In addition, children and adolescents with OCD may try to hide their symptoms due to fear of being mocked or humiliated for their silliness. Another major challenge in identifying OCD in children and adolescents lies in their hesitation in sharing their underlying worries and problems. OCD symptoms often manifest indirectly in children as contrasted with adults. Therefore, it becomes more important for you to be aware of some of the signs that could be indicative of an underlying OCD in the child or adolescent.

| Warning Signs of OCD in Children and Adolescents Given by Danserau & Bouchard (2005) |
|---|
| • Avoiding touching door knobs; use of tissues or handkerchiefs when opening doors. |
| • Seeking repeated reassurance from others through excessive questioning. |
| • Repeated questioning for permission to leave the classroom to go to the lavatory. |
| • Repeated checking of doors, windows, light switches, or written material. |
| • Repeated and/or stereotypical reading of words, text passages or pages in books. |
| • Repeated writing, erasing and overwriting of letters, numbers or words. |
| • Repeated and/or symmetric circling of items in multiple-choice tasks. |
| • Avoidance of contact with sticky substances. |
| • Repeated ordering and arranging items (in an exact symmetrical way). |
| • Repeated and/or ritualized touching of items. |

It is important to realize that, while most adults with OCD would be able to recognize that their thoughts or behaviours are unreasonable, most children would not have such an understanding, thus, making them more resistant to seeking help and also making it difficult to treat the problem. Therefore, the responsibility of identification of OCD in children weighs more heavily on the shoulders of the adults and requires early identification.

## What causes obsessive-compulsive disorder?

As is for most mental health problems, there is no one causative factor that can be singled out for OCD. However, research studies implicate the role of a combined interaction of various genetic, biological and psychosocial factors in the aetiology of OCD.

*Genetic factors:*

OCD has a strong genetic component, being a major contributing factor towards OCD in children. Research studies report that parents, siblings and children of a person with OCD have a greater chance of developing OCD than someone with no family history of the disorder does.

*Biological factors:*

As the role of certain neurotransmitters associated with symptoms of anxiety has been clearly established, research has also demonstrated a link between OCD and insufficient levels of neurotransmitters like serotonin.

*Psychosocial factors:*

Many psychological and social stressors may contribute to the onset and maintenance of OCD such as traumatic events, loss of a loved one, difficulties in relationships, family instability, to name a few. Inconsistent parenting styles and practices, high levels of expressed emotions in the family, experience of abuse or bullying have also been found to be contributory to the development of the disorder.

## Why is early intervention important?

Having an obsessive-compulsive disorder can be one of the most distressing experiences for any individual, and undeniably more so for children and adolescents. It is very difficult for a child to understand his thoughts may be incorrect and he does not have to listen to his mind which is either repeating those thoughts or telling him to repeat actions. Explaining to a child the need to avoid engaging in repetitions is a challenge and the greater the delay in treatment the more rigid the thoughts and actions become, making them difficult to change and treat. Hence, an early intervention cannot be emphasized enough.

The earlier onset of OCD tends to be suggestive of a more chronic and long-term course of the illness, with the obsessive and compulsive symptoms getting more deeply ingrained into the person's belief system and personality. In fact, the sooner an intervention is implemented, the child would be able to develop the right skills, coping mechanisms and support systems and get the correct medical treatment to take care of the illness at an early stage.

Research has shown that suicidal thoughts occur at some point in about as many as half of the individuals with OCD, with suicide attempts being reported up to one-quarter of the individuals with OCD (American Psychological Association, 2013).[6] Furthermore, children and adolescents who have been diagnosed with OCD are at higher risk for developing other comorbid conditions such as depression, or other mood or anxiety disorders, thereby increasing the risk.

For these reasons, it is imperative to stop this cycle at the earliest through early identification and adequate psychiatric and psychological intervention.

### Who is at risk?

Besides the above mentioned aetiological factors that interact together to contribute to the development of OCD in children and adolescents, there are certain other factors that tend to increase the risk of a child developing OCD.

---

[6]The topic of Suicide and Self-Harm is discussed in detail in chapter 20.

> **Red Flags (Beware As These Increase Risk)**
> - Parent with a history of OCD or other psychiatric illness.
> - Anxious, insecure, or perfectionistic disposition.
> - Difficult and challenging family circumstances.
> - History of childhood abuse—verbal, physical, or sexual.
> - Low sense of self.
> - Low peer group support and other support mechanisms.
> - Greater behavioural inhibition in childhood.

The FSMH steps

## STEP 1: Identify the children at risk

You should be on the lookout for any behavioural manifestations of the signs and symptoms of OCD. Besides the warning signs listed previously, given by Danserau and Bouchard in 2005, the following are additional factors you should observe:

- Avoidance of specific situations, places, or people.
- Inability to take simple decisions, feeling confused and unsure.
- Slowness in completing tasks.
- Frequent temper tantrums if not allowed to get own way.
- Need to rigidly stick to rituals and routines.
- Expressing hopelessness or helplessness.
- Drop in grades and class performance.
- Disinterested in being with peers, preferring to be alone.
- Appearing to be engaged in continuous thinking and seeming preoccupied.
- Increased frequency of fights or misunderstandings with peers and others.

## STEP 2: Talk to the child

- **Don't hesitate to begin the conversation and reach out to the child.** When you have identified a child with obsessive-compulsive disorder, it would be difficult to help the child understand what is happening. They may not want to admit that there is a problem and may want to avoid it entirely for fear of embarrassment. It is of great value to help such a child by talking to him, helping him realize that someone does understand and there is a way of explaining the problems they are having. Thus, you should approach the child showing your genuine concern, and at the same time demonstrate your understanding of the nature of the child's problems.
- **Be mindful to generate a rapport first to encourage disclosure.** Children with OCD are likely to be defensive, and therefore it is very important for you to be able to garner the child's trust. The child has been struggling with his inner conflicts for some time now, and he would most likely avoid talking about them. Therefore, it is important for the child to develop a rapport and a trusting relationship with you so that disclosure of problems happens and the child is able to let go of the embarrassment he may experience in discussing them.
- **Be non-confrontational.** Children who have exhibited compulsive behaviour are likely to have been ticked off by the few people who might have noticed their behaviour, being thought of as stubborn and rigid, and may even have been teased or mocked. Such children and adolescents would be likely to experience a low sense of self, at times harbouring the feeling that they do not even deserve to be helped. An empathetic and non-confrontational approach with the child is needed, to be able to express your concerns and demonstrate your support and availability to the child.

## STEP 3: Talk to parents/caregivers

Having identified an obsessive-compulsive child or teenager, it is important to inform the caregivers. An integral part of working with a child who has this problem is involving the family in the treatment process. That is possible only once they have been enlisted into the same by ensuring that their questions are answered, their doubts are clarified, and any misconceptions are removed. Your role in this regard is indispensable.

| Busting Myths Related to OCD in Children and Adolescents |
| --- |
| **OCD is only about being neat and clean** |
| Preoccupations with cleanliness and orderliness are only some types of obsessions and compulsions that people with OCD exhibit. Others including counting, checking, hoarding, doubts and ruminating are also prominently seen. |
| **Stress leads to OCD** |
| While stressful situations do play a major role in the exacerbation as well as maintenance of OCD, stress alone cannot lead to the development of the illness without the presence of other aetiological factors and a neurotransmitter imbalance. |
| **Obsessions and compulsions can be controlled by willpower** |
| OCD is a psychiatric illness, with underlying biological and neuro-chemical changes. Such obsessive thoughts are intrusive, and distressing to the person, and cannot be overcome simply by exerting willpower. |
| **Children cannot have OCD** |
| OCD is a recognized medical illness, which can have an early onset in childhood. In fact, according to NIMH (2013), one-third of adults with OCD had developed the symptoms in their childhood. |

> **OCD cannot be treated; it becomes a part of the personality**
> Successful treatment of OCD involves a combination of pharmacological as well as psychotherapeutic approaches. Moreover, every person with OCD does not necessarily develop an obsessive-compulsive personality.

## STEP 4: Encourage help-seeking and provide information to the family

OCD is a condition which requires proactive treatment. Early intervention is a must as the longer the condition is left untreated it becomes progressively worse, impacting various aspects of the child's life and causing significant impairment. Some of the aspects which you must keep in consideration while working with the family include the following:

- Once the families are able to understand the condition in itself and are able to view it as a factor which can cause significant interference with the child's everyday life, **they must be encouraged consistently to seek treatment**.
- **Families also need to be consistently reminded to not become a part of the child's rituals**. Unknowingly, frequently families start aiding a child in maintaining their rituals, particularly in the initial phases when the illness has just begun and there is not sufficient understanding of this being a medical problem. Before these patterns become too rigid, it would be helpful if families are aided in disengaging from indulging in these behavioural rituals.
- An equally important part is their **persistence with the treatment as the duration for it can be long**. Frequently, once families have witnessed an abating of the symptoms they may wish to withdraw treatment prematurely.

Your role is very pertinent in this regard as it is important that families strictly follow the guidelines and the advice of their psychiatrists.

## STEP 5: Encourage the child to refrain from compulsive behaviour

Frequently, children find it difficult to control their thoughts and impulses to engage in a compulsive act. As the adult around the child who is closely associated with him, it would be helpful if you are able to provide him with support and encouragement in refraining from the same without being too forceful about it. The subtle reminders and reassurances from an adult, who is not family, can help the child in following through with what is being suggested by the experts working with the child.

## STEP 6: Build resilience post the intervention

An illness like OCD after abating would have interfered with various aspects of the child's life in many significant ways. It would have affected daily routines, friendships and relationships, confidence, and the child's sense of self. In such a scenario, your role as the watchful adult involves enabling the reintegration of the child into his old routines and ways of being in his newly changed form. Taking care of the environment surrounding the child is extremely important. Some things that you can do to help the child include the following:

- **Do not overtly treat the child any different** from the others.
- Every child spends maximum time in the school or in the community where you would be a part of his life. **The clinician working with him would need your invaluable inputs** to ensure that every aspect of the problem is taken care of.
- **Be vigilant and observant** and if you notice any signs

of the child returning to previous maladaptive behaviour or responses in the form of obsessions or compulsions, be quick to refer the child back to the treating psychiatrist.
- **Encourage the child with positive reinforcement**, to help him perform in the same way that he used to previously.
- **Emphasize establishing an active support system for the child**, helping him build good relationships with friends and family.
- **Help the child build more effective coping mechanisms by increasing awareness of their own thoughts and feelings, and proactively responding to their inner conflicts**. The child must be encouraged to be expressive and not hesitate to ask for help.
- **Do not get discouraged if the child does not respond appreciatively to your efforts**. Hopelessness and emotional disturbance is part of the illness and usually dissipates with time if proper treatment is being provided.
- **Maintain contact with the child's parents** to ensure that regular and consistent follow-ups are being done post-intervention as well and that things discussed previously are being continued with.

Repetitive and intrusive thoughts and actions that you may have noticed in a child can be an indicant towards the existence of the illness, requiring your urgent attention and intervention. Obsessive-compulsive disorder can become a significant debilitating condition over time, making it essential that it be treated at the earliest.

# 10
# SOMATIC SYMPTOMS AND RELATED DISORDERS

Children often complain about a number of physical problems like stomach aches, headaches, fatigue, breathing difficulties and coughs that seem to aggravate when they experience stress. Sometimes, these symptoms can also mimic neurological disorders like seizures, tremors and paralysis. When these physical complaints cannot be explained by a medical condition, you might be looking at somatic symptom disorders. These are a kind of illnesses that highlight the mind-body connection, where what goes on in one's mind can affect the way our body functions. Of these disorders, **conversion disorder** is the most noteworthy among children and we shall discuss it here.

## Understanding conversion disorder

Conversion disorder is characterized by a symptom or a deficit in voluntary motor or sensory functions. Paralysis, blindness and mutism are the most commonly observed symptoms of conversion.

The hallmark of this condition is that the symptoms cannot be fully explained by a medical cause, and are not intentionally produced. Instead, its root cause is psychological. Even if there is a physical problem, the severity of the suffering cannot be explained by this problem. However, this does not mean that the symptoms are being faked or 'made up' by the child or the adolescent. The pain and suffering of the child are just as real as if they were caused by an actual medical problem. The key aspect of this disorder is the clear presence of a stressor before the onset of the symptom.

As someone interacting and working with children regularly, you must keep in mind that frequent or unexplained medical complaints can be a sign of a psychological distress, which the child may not have verbally expressed. In fact, children with such symptoms often suffer from depression or anxiety and may be grappling with interpersonal problems. How parents and caregivers look at these illnesses determines when and what kind of help is sought.

## Facts

- 68 per cent of children who seek medical treatment have psychological factors associated with their complaints (Rikert & Jay, 1994).
- The onset of conversion disorder is generally from late childhood to early adulthood, and is infrequent before the age of 10.

## How can you identify conversion disorder?

As a caregiver, it can be quite disconcerting to attribute a child's physical symptoms to psychological distress. The diagnosis of conversion disorder, however, can be made if and ONLY if all medical causes have first been investigated and ruled out.

Once all medical conditions have been ruled out, the possibility of conversion disorder needs to be considered. The onset of symptoms is more often than not preceded by a stressful event (such as illness or death of a loved one, academic failure, moving to another school or locality, or abuse).

Typically, the child's complaints will be vague and inconsistent, and not exactly match any specific medical condition. They may describe their illness in a very emotional or dramatic fashion, and may not be able to give the exact sequence of how their symptoms began. In fact, the child will never hurt or harm themselves as a result of a symptom. For example, an adolescent who is suffering from conversion blindness will not fall and hurt himself, or a child who has a psychogenic cough will stop coughing while answering a question or at night while sleeping.

Often, children might exhibit symptoms similar to what they see around them in their family. For instance, a child whose parent had undergone surgery for stomach cancer might develop a stomach ache as his primary physical symptom.

| Warning Signs of Conversion Disorder |
| --- |
| • Experience of sudden blindness |
| • Sudden paralysis |
| • Not being able to speak |
| • Not being able to control movement |
| • Sudden hearing loss |
| • Sudden weakness in the body |
| • Loss of sense of balance |

## What causes conversion disorder?

Various factors have been implicated in the development and emergence of conversion disorder. The following are some of the aspects which are seen as causative factors.

*Biological factors:*

Genetics is known to play a significant role in the emergence of conversion disorder. It is seen more frequently in women than in men.

*Psychological factors:*

Conversion can be viewed as a means of communicating feelings or conflicts that might otherwise be difficult to express. In such a scenario, internal conflicts and anxieties are 'converted' into physical symptoms in a symbolic fashion. Children may benefit from the presence of these symptoms such as getting more attention or favours from others, not having to fulfil roles, tasks or responsibilities and being excused from social obligations or academic expectations. Further, it is possible that children experiencing these symptoms may additionally have low moods and fears or worries as well. This makes it essential that the varied aspects of a child who is suspected of having conversion disorder be explored fully to determine if there are any significant stressors or emotional experiences which have remained unresolved.

*Social factors:*

Observation and learning also play a critical role in the development of conversion. It is a known fact that parental teaching, parental example and ethnic mores can teach some children to demonstrate symptoms of conversion more than others. Typically, the symptoms children and adolescents manifest are those that they have learnt about in the past, mostly from watching other sick members in their family.

## Why is early intervention important?

Conversion disorder is a sign of psychological distress that reflects that the child has learnt an unhealthy or maladaptive way of coping with stressful situations, which can affect the child even in his later years as it would not allow him to seek better ways of solving or resolving a situation. Symptoms can become a potential way of gaining attention and avoiding difficult life situations which would not allow the child to solve the problem effectively. Conversion can also point to the coexistence of other psychiatric conditions such as depression and anxiety, as well as difficulties in interpersonal relationships. Finally, since the complaints are of a physical nature, children may miss out on school and experience academic difficulties which can increase the pressure on them to do well. As a result, intervening early on during the course of the illness is important post the understanding that there is no medical cause for the symptoms being observed.

### Who is at risk?

The life situations a child goes through and his ability and manner of coping with these situations determines the susceptibility to conversion disorder. Some of the factors that have been identified as those that can predispose a child to conversion disorder include those listed in the box below.

> **Red Flags (Beware As These Increase Risk)**
> - History of abuse (physical, emotional, or sexual) or trauma.
> - Being a victim of bullying.
> - Major childhood illness.
> - Poor ability to express emotions.
> - Loss of a loved one.
> - Coexistence of depression or anxiety.

## The FSMH steps

### Step 1: Identify the symptoms of conversion

Physical symptoms of conversion disorder may manifest in the form of any of the following. However, this is not an exhaustive list of symptoms, but rather, the symptoms seen most commonly among children with such problems.

- Involuntary movements and tics
- Seizures
- Abnormal gait and falling
- Falling
- Paralysis
- Weakness
- Blindness and tunnel vision
- Deafness
- Psychogenic vomiting
- Urinary retention
- Diarrhoea

The first step towards intervention for conversion disorder is to refer the child for a medical check-up to eliminate any medical cause. Diagnosis of conversion disorder can only be made after all relevant medical conditions have been ruled out, or if the presence of a medical condition does not explain the extent and severity of the problem.

### Step 2: Look for the triggering stressor

In order for a child to have conversion disorder, it is imperative for there to be a preceding stressor. If you are suspecting the disorder, it is important for you as the adult working with the

---

[7]Identifying depression and anxiety have been dealt with in detail in chapters 4 and 6, respectively.

child to talk to him, his peers, as well as his family to ascertain if the child has been experiencing any kind of conflict or stress or has undergone a trauma of any kind. Also explore for any underlying conditions such as depression or anxiety.[7]

## Step 3: Treat the child's problem as a genuine concern and work towards relieving the symptoms by developing a better understanding

It is the inability to express their emotions verbally that most often leads individuals to somatise, and this is all the more the case when it comes to children and adolescents. The following aspects should be kept in mind while working with the child:

- **Do not neglect the child's suffering.** Just because there is no medical explanation to a symptom does not mean that the child is not suffering. Do not let the child feel that you don't believe him or think that he is making things up. Remember that conversion is a cry for help. Respect what the child is going through and talk to him in an open and non-judgemental manner.

- **Focus on emotions, rather than on the symptom.** When somatizing, it is the symptom that becomes the focus of attention, while the emotions that give rise to it fade into the background. Physical symptoms arise because the child finds it difficult to express their emotions directly. So, in your conversation, try moving beyond the obvious physical complaint and try to understand the child better. Talk to him about his experiences, his friends, and his family and establish an emotional connection.

## Step 4: Use art material and other forms of creative material to communicate

Children who have difficulties expressing themselves verbally might respond better to more creative modes such as art, music, or movement. Additionally, children frequently do not have the vocabulary to be able to express their feelings. It is often seen that a child when asked about his feelings may respond with a shrug of the shoulders or a statement of 'I don't know', which can leave the adult in the situation unsure of what may be happening or whether something is happening or not. In such a scenario, depending on the comfort level of the child, using alternate methods and mediums may encourage self-expression as it would neutralize the situation, act as a distractor or allow for the use of metaphors in art and even allow for the disclosure of difficult material verbally due to a significant level of comfort built in the course of the interactions.

## Step 5: Encourage help-seeking and provide information

Conversion can be difficult to truly comprehend, especially if a doctor concludes that the child is 'fine'. It's, therefore, crucial for you as you work with the child to be able to provide parents/caregivers with the necessary information regarding the condition. Emphasize the point that the child's symptom is not 'nothing'. The child's suffering is real and must be addressed. However, the root cause of this suffering is psychological, rather than biological. In collaboration with the parent, try to explore the stressors and experiences the child may have gone through to develop such a condition. Keep in mind that if you suspect that a child is being abused, it must be reported to the parents and the authorities at the earliest.

At the same time, assess the advantages the child gains by

being sick—is there something he is getting out of it, which might reinforce the sick behaviour. Once sure of the diagnosis, encourage the parents to modify the environment at home to ensure that the child is not getting any undue advantages by virtue of being 'sick'. Removing such reinforcements can go a long way in managing this condition.

Children suffering from conversion disorder require professional intervention. Medical intervention in the form of psychiatric medication can also be required, which should be communicated to the family and caregivers. Encourage caregivers to consult a psychologist to help the child deal with his conflicts and cope better with stress.

### Busting Myths Related to Conversion Disorder

#### Children cannot develop conversion disorder

Although considered to be rare, conversion disorder in children is generally seen to have an onset from late childhood to early adulthood. Developmentally, typical young patients can have apparent paresis without a demonstrated physiological cause for a few hours or days after a minor injury. Difficulty expressing emotional distress verbally is widely thought to underlie the presentation of physical symptoms that cannot be explained in medical terms.

#### Children fake conversion disorder symptoms to escape responsibilities

Children diagnosed with conversion disorder often experience their body functions in distressing and disturbing ways, just as someone with an underlying structural abnormality would experience it. Common symptoms experienced by children that may be expressed in response to unresolved stress include headache, dizziness, abdominal pain, tinnitus, ataxia, generalized weakness, focal weakness, paresthesia, blurry vision, vision loss, tunnel vision, and non-epileptic seizures.

> **Conversion disorder is indicative of abuse of the child**
> Physical and sexual abuse has been reported in some cases of conversion disorder in children. However, other causes include stressors such as school difficulties, bullying, the death of a loved one (including pets!), or parental divorce. Abuse in itself is not the only cause for conversion disorder in children.

## Step 6: Build resilience post the intervention

The necessary psychological treatment can go on for a while. However, there are some adjustments that must be made to the child's social environment during and after the treatment as well:

- **Do not treat the child differently from others.** As mentioned before, social benefits and advantages can reinforce the child's condition. Make sure that the child is not cut any slack, or given any leeway on account of his symptoms.
- **Provide a warm and supportive environment** where children are able to share and discuss comfortably whatever it is that is bothering them. Allowing for and encouraging free expression without any fear of criticism or ridicule are essential.
- **Help the child come up with better strategies for coping with stress.** Partner with the child to brainstorm effective solutions to problems and practice them with the child, be it for their studies or their personal relationships. Role-playing these solutions is usually found to be very beneficial in such a situation.
- **Reassure the child about the safety of the current environment.** A child who has been a victim of trauma and abuse and who is displaying symptoms of conversion would need continued reassurance of the safety of the environment that he is currently in. Engage in this only if you are certain about the safety of the child's environment as it is very

important for the child to be able to continue to trust you.
- **Maintain regular contact with the parents** to ensure that the child's home environment is relatively stress-free and that consistent follow-ups are being done with the psychologist for therapy.
- **Stay connected with the treating external professionals.** The external experts would be getting a lot of inputs from the child which would be helpful to you and would also benefit from your inputs regarding his real environmental situation. This reciprocity of information sharing is crucial for the child to be able to overcome the conversion disorder.

The presence of conversion disorder can be easily missed given the manner in which the symptoms mimic those of physical health conditions. The presence of conversion disorder indicates the need to explore the situations surrounding the child's life to help him develop the vocabulary to be able to share the problem and cope with stressors effectively.

# 11
# ATTENTION-DEFICIT/HYPERACTIVITY DISORDER

Many children occasionally forget their homework, have trouble maintaining focus on the task at hand, act without thinking, or get fidgety and restless when required to sit at one place. As adults who work with children, you would have commonly observed children who just can't seem to sit still, who never seem to listen, who can't follow instructions no matter how clearly you present them, or who blurt out inappropriate comments at inappropriate times. Often these children are labelled as 'lazy' or 'troublemakers', are criticized for making careless mistakes and are seen as being disobedient, frequently getting screamed at or punished for the errors they make which tend to be quite repetitive and make you feel that they just don't listen when something is said or explained to them. These children might have an **attention-deficit/hyperactivity disorder**.

A child with **attention-deficit/hyperactivity disorder (ADHD)**[8] would exhibit a pattern of inattention and/or hyperactivity-impulsivity that would significantly interfere with his academic, social as well as daily functioning. It is important to

---

[8] A child with ADHD can present with either inattentive behaviour, or with hyperactivity-impulsivity, or even a combination of both.

note that such inattentiveness and hyperactivity is commonly seen in many children. But what stands out in a child with ADHD is that he would persistently display such a pattern of behaviour for at least six months. This pattern is developmentally inappropriate, typically being observed during school years before the age of 12. Furthermore, such behaviour would be displayed not just in school but also at home, or in other settings as well.

A child's **inattentive behaviour** typically manifests in the form of the following:

- Easy distractibility
- Carelessness
- Forgetfulness
- Inability to work at a single task for a sustained period of time
- Frequently leaving tasks unfinished
- Not seeming to listen even when spoken to directly
- Often not following instructions
- Difficulties in organizing tasks

On the other hand, **hyperactivity and impulsivity** in children could include the following manifestations in their behaviour:

- Appearing to be constantly 'on the go'
- Excessive fidgeting or squirming
- Frequently leaving the seat
- Talking non-stop
- Unable to do anything quietly
- Impatience
- Frequently interrupting or intruding

### Facts

- ADHD is by far one of the most common yet grossly misunderstood disorders that are found in children.
- The prevalence rates for ADHD are estimated to be between

5 to 10 per cent of the general population in India (Malhi & Singhi, 2000).
- ADHD is five times more likely to occur in boys rather than girls (Malhi & Singhi, 2000).

**Identifying ADHD**

Being able to differentiate between ADHD and normal behaviour in children is important as frequently children can come across as being either restless or inattentive. It is the persistence of these problems for at least six months and their presence in multiple settings which is an important aspect in distinguishing them. Besides these two aspects the following are the warning signs which could indicate the presence of a problem.

| Warning Signs for ADHD ||
|---|---|
| Inattention | Hyperactivity-Impulsivity |
| • Difficulty in doing any activity at length | • Unable to sit still |
| • Making careless mistakes | • Fidgety and restless |
| • Often misplacing belongings | • Always running around |
| • Daydreaming | • Cannot wait for their turn |
| • Leaving work unfinished | • Appears disobedient |
| • Avoiding work that requires attention | • Interrupts others |
| • Starts tasks but gets sidetracked | • Acts without thinking |
| • Difficulty in meeting deadlines | • Always energetic |
| • Forgetful even in daily routine activities | • Disruptive behaviour |

## What causes ADHD?

There is no exact cause of ADHD which has been identified as yet. Although it is hypothesized that a combination of many factors interacts to play a role in ADHD, today it is primarily recognized as a neurological disorder.

*Genetic factors:*

ADHD tends to run in families. Studies have shown certain genetic characteristics that occur with high frequency in families where one or more family member has ADHD. Researchers are in the process of identifying the genes that can be implicated in the causation of ADHD.

*Birth and delivery related conditions:*

A child could develop a susceptibility to ADHD since the time of conception itself. Previous research has shown that there is a strong link between the mother's health during pregnancy and the development of ADHD. Furthermore, prenatal exposure to toxic substances can also have an effect on the developing brain tissues, thereby leading to sustained behavioural issues such as hyperactivity in later life. Children who have suffered a brain injury in infancy may also show some behaviour similar to those of ADHD such as inattention, poor regulation of motor activity and impulsivity.

## Why is early intervention important?

In the light of the problems that come associated with a diagnosis of ADHD, early identification is of undeniable importance. The sooner a child is identified, the better are the chances of a successful treatment. Moreover, inattention and hyperactivity-impulsivity symptoms, if persisting into adulthood, could lead to significant long-term impairments in the individual's academic, social, emotional as well as occupational functioning.

ADHD is often comorbid with other disorders as well such as depression, learning disability, oppositional or conduct disorder and early intervention becomes all the more imperative in these cases. Due to underachievement in academics on account of the difficulty in paying attention or the restlessness and hyperactivity the child experiences, children with ADHD are also at a risk for failure at school and dropout. They might be ridiculed and teased by their peers due to the difficulties they face and the trouble they get into with adults. Bullying is also found to be associated with ADHD children, where they can be either a victim or a bully. Also, these children are more likely to indulge in risk-taking behaviour like early experimentation with drugs, sexual activity and altercations with authority. Therefore, it is essential to ensure an earlier identification to enable adequate intervention as soon as possible. This would provide the foundation so that the child is able to perform to the best of his ability and potential.

## Who is at risk?

There are certain factors that have been identified to implicate a higher risk for the child or adolescent to develop ADHD.

| Red Flags (Beware As These Increase Risk) |
|---|
| • History of ADHD in the family.<br>• Exposure to toxic substances before or during infancy.<br>• Obstetrical complications during pregnancy. |

## The FSMH steps

### STEP 1: Identify the children at risk

An integral role while working with children is to be able to identify the behaviour which could signal that the child has ADHD. In addition to the warning signs and features mentioned previously, some common examples of the behaviour you need to observe include the following:

- Poor relationship with peers on account of behaviour problems
- Underachiever despite being bright or intelligent
- Disrupting the classroom
- 'Lazy' or 'troublemaker'
- Frequent complaints by teachers/parents
- Always in motion
- Appearing to be lost in thoughts
- Cluttered and untidy
- Difficult to control
- Frequently overlooking details
- Experiences difficulty in planning and in being organized
- Frequently loses things
- Gets into fights
- Is easily injured
- Does not show consequential thinking

## STEP 2: Work with the child sensitively and patiently

- **Take the initiative to begin a conversation.** If you believe that you have identified a child who might be at risk for ADHD, it is a good idea for you to address the child directly. Considering the importance of early identification, you should not hesitate to take the initiative, as these children need someone to talk to them about their behaviour, to help them understand what they are doing, and how they can be helped.
- **Remember that you need to be patient.** The child with ADHD would need a lot of careful and considered handling.

You would need to be extremely patient working with the child. It would be important to maintain your sense of calm as there would be several moments when you would feel challenged and frustrated as the child may not be able to follow all instructions easily.

- **Be non-confrontational in your interactions with the child.** Children with ADHD would be accustomed to being scolded or punished for their laziness or their disobedience. Therefore, it is important for you to be able to communicate with the child in a non-confrontational manner, to allow their experience to be relaxed and calm as compared to their conflicts with other authority figures. Redirect the blame from the child to the illness and symptoms that are associated with the illness.
- **Break down instructions for the child.** While working with the child, break down your instructions to him into simple and easy steps. This would help ensure that the child is able to follow through with each activity to completion since a significant part of the problem for the child is being able to stay focused on a task for long and they can forget to take activities through to completion if they have too many steps associated with them.
- **Be empathetic.** You are the responsible adult whom the child is trusting, and you need to show your genuine concern for the child. Try to understand the child's difficulties and experiences. Usually, children with ADHD have many social issues as well in terms of being unable to connect with a peer group—bullying, teasing and social isolation besides dealing with academic difficulties. They are often misunderstood by authority figures and can be distrustful of them. Therefore, it is important that you make yourself accessible to the child and encourage him to talk about his experiences.
- **Provide reassurance.** Children with ADHD would have faced disappointments and failures, and might even feel

helpless. It is very important to address their emotional and psychological concerns as they may not be adept at expressing themselves. These children can often have associated problems like low self-esteem, self-blame, anger or aggression and early experimentation with substance use. Reassure the child by providing him information about the illness and help him formulate better strategies to deal with the problems he is experiencing.

## STEP 3: Inform the parent/caregiver

Often parents would overlook the symptoms of ADHD as signs of laziness or being extremely troublesome, assuming that the child would improve and show changes with age. Once you have identified a child you suspect of being at risk for ADHD, and requires a formal assessment by a mental health professional, you would first need to inform the parents. Parents typically find it difficult to accept the possibility of a clinical condition in their child. It can be an anxiety-provoking situation for the parent, especially when ADHD as a disorder is shrouded in misconception and lack of awareness. Therefore, it is very important for parents to be well-informed of such issues so that proper treatment and care can be provided to the child.

- **Demonstrate your understanding and address fears.** As important as it is to talk to the child and provide reassurance, it is equally important to understand a parent's emotional and psychological state while talking to them about their child. It is useful to acknowledge their fears through a simple reflection like, 'I can understand your concern, being a parent it is natural for you to feel this way.' To have someone address one's emotion can be very calming. Make sure that you show empathy at all times. This will help in making the parent more receptive towards the communication.
- **Do not label.** When talking about the child, do not appear

to be critical of the problems the child has been experiencing as this only serves to put the parent on the defensive. Talk about both strengths as well as weaknesses of the child, by beginning with the child's positives. It is important to not label the child, but rather to focus on the problematic behaviour and ways to solve them. Ask the parent if they face similar behavioural issues with the child at home and what strategies they have tried to deal with the same. Listen to their problems and perspectives carefully and respectfully.
- **Bust myths.** Not many parents would understand the meaning and connotation of ADHD and may harbour many myths. Psycho-educating the parents about the nature of the illness can help in busting such myths.

| Busting Myths Related to ADHD |
|---|
| **ADHD is a label for bad behaviour** |
| ADHD is an identifiable neurobiological condition that affects children all over the world. It requires timely intervention or it may lead to more severe behavioural, emotional and academic difficulties. It is not a label for bad behaviour. |
| **ADHD is only seen in boys** |
| While ADHD is more commonly diagnosed amongst boys, girls also exhibit such behaviour. This misconception is probably rooted in the more common display of hyperactivity by males. Moreover, as symptoms of inattention are less obvious than symptoms of hyperactivity, girls may not be diagnosed as often or as much. |
| **Children automatically outgrow ADHD** |
| Until recently it was believed that ADHD did not continue into adolescence, based on the assumption that hyperactivity often diminishes during the teen years. However, we now know that many symptoms of ADHD can continue into adulthood, causing significant long-term impairments in behavioural, social, cognitive and academic functioning. |

| **ADHD children cannot attend regular school** |
|---|
| ADHD has no relationship with a child's intelligence. They are just as bright as children without ADHD. However, such children require the special attention of teachers and parents alike, with specific behavioural principles being tailored to their needs to ensure that their symptoms do not interfere in their own or other children's learning. They can easily attend regular school like all other children of their age. |
| **Bad parenting causes ADHD** |
| ADHD is not what happens when parents fail to keep their child in check or teach them good behaviour. Parents are in no way responsible for their child having ADHD. When a child with ADHD blurts things out or gets out of his seat in class, it is not because he has not been taught that such behaviour is wrong. It is because he cannot control his impulses. However, parents play a major role in the treatment and management process. |
| **An ADHD child is doomed to fail** |
| Given the right kind of intervention, treatment and opportunity, children with ADHD can overcome their difficulties and rise to great heights. |

## STEP 4: Give basic behaviour management tips to the parents

Parents of the child with ADHD experience significant difficulties in managing his behaviour and helping him with his academic curriculum. This can lead to conflict between the parent and the child and it would be important for you to help resolve this conflict as early as possible even before treatment by a professional begins. Some of the things which would aid in taking care of this aspect include the following:

- **Help parents to understand that shouting, screaming, hitting or excessive punishment will not help** in bringing about change in the child's behaviour.

- **Encourage parents to be patient** and if they feel incapable of controlling their anger then they should distance themselves from the child first, calm down and then address the problem.
- **Encourage parents to see the child's strengths** as well and not focus only on his problem areas.
- **Help them break instructions into small parts** to ensure that the child does not forget or get distracted from the task.
- **Encourage parents to give the child frequent breaks** in order to ensure that he does not experience a sense of boredom while engaging in tasks.

## STEP 5: Be cognizant of other problems the child may be experiencing

- A hallmark of ADHD is its potential to create problems for the child in multiple areas. Be aware that besides having the problems of hyperactivity, impulsivity or easy distractibility, **the child may also experience challenges in academics, in maintaining relationships, in solving problems, or having consequential thinking, being bullied or bullying others, or getting angry and aggressive**. It is your knowledge of these which would form the cornerstone of ensuring that treatment accorded to the child is able to take care of all aspects of his functioning and is not restrictive in nature. The emotional distress of the child must never be neglected.
- The experience of ADHD can be a difficult one and **the child needs a non-judgemental outlet to be able to express his feelings**. Encourage the child to understand and express his emotions through any medium that he is comfortable with—art, journaling, writing, or music.
- Along with behaviour therapy, **social-skills training is also important to enable the child to form sustainable peer relationships and to enhance the acceptability and self-**

**esteem of the child**. This means making sure that situations where the child may be bullied or harassed are minimized and the child is not reprimanded in full public view.
- **Parents and teachers should be encouraged to tailor their teaching strategies to meet the needs of the child.** Efforts can be made to help them by using more visual aids to enhance their attention capacities, and make it easier for them to grasp newer concepts.
- **It is very important to maintain regular contact with the parent and monitor the treatment.** Creating a partnership between home and school is important to ensure consistency and the effectiveness in the learning of adaptive behaviour and in this respect your role would be irreplaceable.

## STEP 6: Build resilience post the intervention

ADHD is one such problem which requires continued and sustained interventions. The nature of this problem makes it imperative that someone be involved to monitor the possible eruption of a problem once the initial intervention has taken place and the primary problems are resolved. This aspect falls squarely within the purview of what you as an adult would need to monitor. The child would require understanding and support and gentle-shaping of his behaviour which is possible only if the problem is fully understood and lofty expectations of sudden changes are not placed upon the child. Patience is a key to working with children with ADHD and the nature of the relationship forged with the child would hold undeniable importance in enabling the process of transformation and change.

# 12
# DISRUPTIVE BEHAVIOUR DISORDERS

It is not unusual for children to be naughty or to even defy authority from time to time. All children at some point display such behaviour which also forms to some degree a part of the developmental process of understanding discipline and boundaries. They may talk back to parents and teachers, argue, question or refuse to obey certain rules and regulations. However, the factors which characterize **disruptive behaviour disorders** are the severity, regularity as well as pervasiveness of such behaviour, and the level of impairment caused on account of the same.

In children with a disruptive behaviour disorder, 'breaking rules' is a regular pattern that may seem to get progressively worse, thereby interfering in the child's ability to function adequately in school as well as at home. They would display persistently problematic behaviour, including breaking and flouting of rules, being aggressive, destructive, troublesome and uncooperative with both peers as well as authority figures. Such behaviour would be significantly greater in their intensity and frequency in comparison to their peers of a similar age group.

**Facts**

- Disruptive behaviour disorders are the most common mental health disorder among children with a rate of 4–9 per cent among all children from birth to 18 years of age, with a prevalence as high as 15 per cent in children and adolescents (*The Merck Manual of Diagnosis and Therapy*, 2011).
- The disruptive behaviour disorders tend to be more common in males than in females, although the relative degree of male predominance may differ both across disorders and within a disorder at different ages (DSM-5, 2014).
- Early patterns of disruptive behaviour may become a lifelong pervasive repertoire culminating in adult antisocial personality disorder (Kaplan and Sadock, 2007).

**Signs and symptoms of disruptive behaviour disorders**

Disruptive behaviour is characterized by a persistent pattern of uncooperative, defiant and hostile behaviour towards peers and/or authority figures that has an adverse impact by interfering with the child's or adolescent's day-to-day functioning. Such behaviour needs to be consistent across more than one setting including home, school, or community. The disruptive behaviour disorders can be considered to be linked to a common externalizing spectrum associated with the personality dimensions labelled as *disinhibition* and (inversely) *constraint* and, to a lesser extent, negative emotionality.

Disruptive behaviour disorders in children could take the form of either an **oppositional defiant disorder (ODD)** or a **conduct disorder (CD)**.

*Oppositional defiant disorder:*

Children with oppositional defiant disorder tend to exhibit a pattern of behaviour which having persisted for at least six months, is characterized by the following:

- Anger or irritability
- Temper outbursts
- Active refusal to comply with rules
- Uncooperative behaviour with both peers as well as adults
- Deliberately annoying behaviour
- Resentful and spiteful behaviour
- Blaming others for their misbehaviour

Such behaviour tend to be in excess of what would be expected of other children of the same age, and typically cause significant amount of distress to other children and adults, especially those familiar with the child or who he is closest to, than to the child himself.

*Conduct disorder:*

Children diagnosed with having conduct-related problems are likely to display a repeated and persistent pattern of behaviour in which the basic rights of others or major age-appropriate societal norms or rules are violated. Typically these problems tend to have persisted for a long time, more than a year to be specific, and they are characterized by the following:

- Aggression and cruelty towards both people and animals.
- Destructive and violent behaviour with others as well as own belongings.
- Stealing and lying behaviour.
- Running away from school or home, before the age of 13.
- Bullying, threatening, or intimidating others.

The primary difference between these two disorders is the severity of disruptive behaviour, as the behaviour of oppositional defiant disorder are typically of a less severe nature than those of conduct disorder. Children with CD are more likely to be aggressive, destructive and deceitful, whereas children with ODD are more likely to be angry or irritable. These disorders may also be considered to be on a progressive continuum, in which case the lack of adequate and timely interventions when signs of ODD are noticed, can cause it to progress to become CD which then might progress to become **Anti-Social Personality Disorder** in adulthood.

## How can you identify disruptive behaviour disorders?

Often, children with disruptive behaviour disorders invariably present maximum misbehaviour in specific settings as compared to others. For instance, parents would frequently report that their child is at his worst behaviour at home, putting on a better face at school or with peers. But others might typically display their misbehaviour outside the home first, later spreading it to the home setting as well. Typically, disruptive behaviour would become evident in any setting in which the child spends a considerable amount of time, and hence, it becomes important for you to be aware of the signs of such misbehaviour which may point towards the onset of a larger problem.

As people working closely with children and adolescents, you should be alert to the following kinds of behaviour which can be warning signs for the onset of disruptive behaviour disorders:

| Warning Signs of Disruptive Behaviour Disorders |
| --- |
| • Excessive complaints from teachers or peers |
| • Disinterest in academics |
| • Poor or irregular attendance |
| • Lack of a consistent set of friends |
| • Befriending children of older age groups or so-called problematic children |

| |
|---|
| • Frequent violations of rules and regulations |
| • Complete disregard for authority figures |
| • Alcohol and substance use |
| • Excessive irritability or anger |

It is also important for you to be aware that children and adolescents with disruptive behaviour are also at risk for suicidal behaviour. Furthermore, adolescents with disruptive behaviour disorders are adept at hiding their misconduct, whereas in some severe cases, they might not even make any attempts to conceal their actions. Moreover, it is not uncommon for such adolescents to indulge in uninhibited sexual behaviour or substance use.

## What causes disruptive behaviour disorders?

There is no single factor that can fully account for a child's disruptive behaviour. Rather, the aetiology of disruptive behaviour disorders is a complex amalgam of several factors including neurological, psychological, social and environmental factors.

*Neurological factors:*

Children with disruptive behaviour may have certain impairments in the functioning of the brain that cause changes in their neurotransmitter levels, which lead to dysregulation of the child's emotional and impulse controls. Abnormalities in the prefrontal cortex and the amygdala have been found to be implicated in children with disruptive behaviour.

*Psychological factors:*

Children who have been brought up in disruptive conditions often learn to use maladaptive coping mechanisms with a poor regulation of their impulses and emotions. Children with strict parenting might lack a sense of empathy having observed hostile environment in their childhood. Other factors like inconsistent parenting styles or being a target of physical violence, negative and harsh verbalizations or a lack of warmth from caregivers also play an instrumental role in the aetiology of disruptive behaviour.

*Social factors:*

Social factors like poverty, a large family size, abuse in the family and early institutionalization have been implicated in playing a causal role in the development of disruptive behaviour. Unemployed parents, lack of a supportive social network, and lack of positive participation in community activities have also been found to predict disruptive behaviour in children and adolescents. It is widely accepted that children chronically exposed to violence, or even witnesses to any form of abuse, may learn to demonstrate disruptive behaviour in the form of aggression and destruction.

*Environmental factors:*

As children are most vulnerable to observing from their surroundings, the impact of media and the environment has a major role to play in determining their behaviour. Moreover, early exposure to violent behaviour in childhood is a major factor responsible for shaping a child's display of disruptive behaviour. Also, the influence of the media cannot be negated, as portrayals of violence have a huge impact on the child. Even videogames that promote violence have been found to play a major role in the development of disruptive behaviour in children and adolescents.

## Why is early intervention important?

The earliest possible intervention in disruptive behaviour is vital because, the sooner such behaviour is identified, the more successful are the chances for its efficient modification.

Considering the high rate of comorbidity among children with disruptive behaviour, including higher risks of having attention-deficit/hyperactivity disorder, substance use, anxiety, mood or other impulse control disorders—it becomes imperative to ensure that they get timely psychiatric and psychological intervention as soon as possible as this disorder becomes progressively difficult to treat, which might eventually culminate into an anti-social personality disorder in adulthood.

## Who is at risk?

While some children are prone to develop disruptive behaviour as maladaptive coping mechanisms, there are certain factors, the presence of which has been identified to implicate and result in a higher risk for the child or adolescent to develop disruptive behaviour disorders.

| Red Flags (Beware As These Increase Risk) |
| --- |
| • Neglectful, harsh, or inconsistent parenting<br>• Association with delinquent peers<br>• Neighbourhood risk<br>• Exposure to violence or abuse<br>• Poor frustration tolerance<br>• History of physical or emotional trauma<br>• Early institutional living<br>• Parental criminality |

## The FSMH steps

### STEP 1: Identify the children at risk

As mentioned above, it is extremely important for you to be on the lookout for the warning signs that could lead to the precipitation of disruptive behaviour disorders so as to ensure early identification and intervention for the problem behaviour. In addition to the warning signs enlisted previously, the following are some behavioural signs that you should be wary of:

- Disregard for instructions
- Often interrupting, intruding, or arguing
- Reckless misbehaviour with disregard for rules
- Lack of fear of consequences
- Frequent physical or verbal fights
- Not listening when spoken to

## STEP 2: Talk to the child you have identified as being at risk

- **Take the initiative to begin a conversation.** A child with a disruptive behaviour disorder will not typically be open to seeking help, usually denying his misbehaviour, providing excessive justifications and blaming it on others. Considering the importance of early identification, you should not hesitate to take the initiative, as these children need someone to talk to them about their behaviour, to help them understand what they are doing, and how they can be helped.
- **Do not be confrontational.** Children and adolescents who have been displaying disruptive behaviour are often habituated to being scolded or punished for their misbehaviour. Therefore it is important for you to be able to communicate with the child in a non-confrontational manner, to allow this experience to be empathetic as compared to being conflictual with other authority figures.
- **Do not label**, as labelling the child as a troublemaker makes the communication appear to be loaded with negativity and resentment. Moreover, it leads us to have assumptions about his behaviour and makes it difficult to see the child as a whole without any biases regarding his strengths and weaknesses. Besides actively listening to and engaging with the child,

it is essential to model appropriate behaviour and to help them realize that your help and support is available to them.
- **Be calm.** While playing the role of the responsible and supportive adult in this relationship, it is important for you to maintain your calm while talking to the child. Children learn through mirroring and observation and you do not want to exacerbate the oppositional traits in the child. So you should avoid being critical, as it could make them defensive as well as defiant. Refrain from using a loud and angry voice, speak calmly and clearly, and make eye contact while controlling your facial expressions, posture and gestures.
- **Focus on the now.** Do not play the blame game with the child or revisit every problem that he has ever been in. Instead, try to use shorter explanations in place of longer lectures. Talk about what is happening right now as this makes the situation more concrete for the child to understand. Focussing on solutions rather than problems and giving regular and positive feedback to the child also go a long way in making the communication effective.

## STEP 3: Inform the parent/caregiver

Once you have identified a child you suspect is displaying disruptive behaviour, it is necessary for you to inform his parents. This can be an extremely challenging task as you run the risk of being completely stonewalled by the parent. No parent would like to acknowledge a problem with their child due to multiple reasons. It can be an anxiety-provoking situation for the parent, especially when a disruptive behaviour disorder is shrouded in misconception and lack of awareness. Such a communication can be perceived as an insult by some parents, and it may come across to some as a lifelong impairment that would dampen the dreams of their child along with their own hopes and aspirations.

As the informer, you may be faced with reactions ranging

from extreme denial and anger to breakdown and panic. There are certain things that you would need to keep in mind when talking about this to the parent or caregiver.

- **Address fears.** It is important to understand a parent's emotional and psychological state while talking to them about their child. It is useful to acknowledge their fears through a simple reflection like, 'This is certainly a difficult situation for you. I understand the worry and anxiety you may be experiencing right now.' To have someone address one's emotional experience can be very calming. Make sure that you show empathy at all times. This will help in making the parent more receptive to the communication.
- **Give complete information.** Incomplete information can create a bigger challenge for your work with the child's parents or caregivers. Providing them with a detailed understanding of the problem, its complexities, the impact it can have, as well as the way forward in terms of the help that they need to seek is essential for enlisting them in the entire journey of the treatment process.
- **Bust myths.** Not many parents would understand the meaning and connotation of disruptive behaviour disorders and may harbour many myths. Psychoeducation about the nature of the illness and the next steps in the intervention also need to be communicated to the parent.

| Busting Myths Related to Disruptive Behaviour Disorders |
|---|
| **Disruptive behaviour disorder is a label given to rebellious behaviour** |
| While it is a fact that all children can be rebellious and difficult to handle from time to time, but not all of them will have a disruptive behaviour disorder. This disorder occurs when the disruptive behaviour is consistent, severe and interferes with the child's relationships at home, in school and in the community. |

**Children with disruptive behaviour just need stricter rules**
Children with disruptive behaviour are extremely confrontational in nature and like to engage in power struggles. Falling into such a struggle where it becomes about one-upmanship based on authority, is going to be counter-productive with such children. Treating a disruptive behaviour disorder is about using consistent rules, along with warmth, care and trust. Both these aspects are equally important.

**Disruptive behaviour disorders are only prevalent in boys**
While a significantly higher number of boys do get diagnosed with disruptive behaviour disorders, girls also do indulge in disruptive behaviour. The ways in which aggression is displayed differs for the genders due to which disruptive behaviour in boys gets more highlighted as compared to girls who often resort to malicious rumours rather than direct violence.

**Children automatically outgrow disruptive behaviour**
As is with any illness—mental or physical—ignoring the problem is never the right answer. Especially for disruptive behaviour, if not given adequate and timely intervention, these children often continue to display worrying behaviour right into adulthood, being at a higher risk of developing anti-social personalities. Without intervention, such children and adolescents often get involved in unlawful activities as well.

## STEP 4: Encourage help-seeking and provide information

After talking to the child and his parents or caregivers, it is also necessary to show them the path forward. You can reassure them by providing the complete and correct information about the various courses of action needed towards intervention.

Disruptive disorders require adequate medical and psychological intervention, and hence the role of professional help is irreplaceable. Intervention with such disruptive behaviour encompasses the clinic, home as well as the school and classroom setting in order to be holistic in nature. Treatment of disruptive behaviour is a long-term process and cannot happen in isolation of the environment that the child is in.

A child with a disruptive behaviour disorder would require training for social skills, self-expression and communication, emotional regulation, behaviour modification and academic training. These are only possible when the parent/caregiver works in close tandem with the teacher, counsellor or the community worker as well as the external professionals.

## STEP 5: Encourage parental involvement

Intervention for disruptive behaviour of children is not possible without the involvement of parents, as the child's behaviour needs to be monitored as well as regulated in all settings. A vital ingredient of a successful behavioural modification is essayed in the application of such interventions consistently. It is important not only for you to be aware of some such interventional strategies, but also to encourage the parents or the caregivers towards their application at home.

- **Use a reward system.** Rewards and reinforcements need to be used wisely, in order to be effective in modifying the child's behaviour. An example of an effective reward system is utilizing token economy, which allows children and adolescents to earn privileges, praise, peer recognition or recognition from parents. It is important to ensure that the reward system is simple and easily understood by the child as well as the parent or caregiver.
- **Use feedback effectively.** It is useful to make the child aware of his own behaviour, and to be given feedback for the same. He must be made to realize the relation between his behaviour as well as the associated consequences. Parents should be encouraged to look out for 'good behaviour' to find opportunities to praise the child as well, instead of

focussing only on misbehaviour.
- **Specifically state rules and consequences.** The child or adolescent must be informed of the set of rules and regulations clearly, with the consequences expected. It is very useful to involve the children in the process of deciding these rules, as it makes them feel more responsible and committed, and also reduces their chances of defiance.
- **Establish boundaries.** Children with disruptive behaviour often lack the understanding of certain social cues that come naturally to the rest of us. They can often be inappropriate without even realizing it. It is important to form very clear boundaries with such a child and this needs to be explained to the parents as well.

## STEP 6: Build resilience post the intervention

The most important factor in the treatment of disruptive behaviour is the maintenance post-intervention. Children with disruptive behaviour typically have had difficulties in maintaining healthy relationships with their peers, and they are prone to face difficulties in rebuilding relationships with the same peer groups. As the individual working closely with the child, it is important for you to remember the following:

- **Do not overtly treat the child any different from the others,** remember that other children will also take cue from you on how to interact and behave with the child.
- **Educate other children about the child's disruptive behaviour**, and the need for them to reciprocate in an encouraging and supporting manner.
- **Work on helping the child build good relationships** with friends and family.
- **Encourage the child's efforts** towards re-establishing better relationships.
- **Help the child negotiate problems and challenges** by

working on problem-solving and decision-making.
- **Encourage the child to engage in more pro-social behaviour.**
- **Use praise and rewards consistently** to bring about an effective change in the child's behaviour.
- **Maintain contact with the parents and if possible with the mental health professional** to ensure that regular and consistent follow-ups are being done with regard to the disruptive behaviour.

## STEP 7: Promote a prevention policy

Studying or living in an environment that is sensitized and oriented towards the needs of the child with disruptive behaviour goes a long way in preventing severe manifestations of the disorder. These children generally come from very inconsistent backgrounds and need to learn the importance of rules and regulations, understanding and managing emotions, and resolving social conflicts. Running schoolwide programmes like life-skills training on anti-bullying, anger management, social-skills training, conflict resolution and peer mediation programs can go a long way in equipping these children with skills to understand themselves better and deal with their aggression and other behaviour problems in a more effective and acceptable manner.

# 13
# EATING DISORDERS

There is an undeniable importance attached to the role of eating food in our lives. Almost all of us do at some point of time eat too much or too little, have cravings, or make efforts to eat more healthy food. There is a two-way relationship between food and mood. Children might lose their appetite when they are stressed, or might resort to comfort eating during exams.

**Eating disorders** refer to such extreme disturbances in eating behaviour, wherein the urge to eat less or more is no more in the person's control, and the person feels distressed about his body weight and shape. Commonly observed habits could include following rigid diets, secretly binging on food, throwing up after meals, using laxatives, excessive exercising, or obsessively counting calories.

## Facts

- Eating disorders are one of the most common psychiatric problems faced by females, having been reported in upto 4 per cent of adolescent and young adult students (Saddock, Saddock & Ruiz, 2015).
- According to the NIMH, eating disorders affect 2.7 per cent of 13 to 17-year-olds worldwide (2010).

- 25–33 per cent of people with anorexia or bulimia nervosa develop a chronic disorder (WHO, 2004).
- However, these disorders are mostly under-reported, and hence adequate and timely help is not always able to reach those who need it. A major hindrance to the timely treatment of the condition is also the lack of awareness, understanding and knowledge which could facilitate timely identification.

## Signs and symptoms of eating disorders

Eating disorders are characterized by a persistent disturbance of eating or eating-related behaviour, which alters the person's consumption or absorption of food, and interferes with the affected individual's health and daily functioning, such as going to school and maintaining relationships with friends and family.

The common symptoms of eating disorders could include behaviour that interferes with weight gain persisting for the past three months, with an average of at least once a week, which could be:

(a) **Restrictive** behaviour including dieting, fasting or excessive exercising, and/or
(b) **Overeating/purging** behaviour including self-induced vomiting, or the misuse of laxatives, diuretics, or enemas.

*Anorexia nervosa:*

In addition to the above mentioned aspects, adolescents with **anorexia nervosa** would also have:

- An intense fear of gaining weight.
- A distorted perception of body shape or weight.
- Trying to maintain body weight that is less than the minimally normal weight required according to their age, gender and development.

*Bulimia nervosa and binge eating disorders:*

Bulimia nervosa and binge eating disorders include overeating. Characteristic aspects of this overeating include the following:

- A feeling that the person cannot stop eating or control what or how much to eat.
- Eating even when not hungry or when feeling uncomfortably full.
- Eating much faster than normal and preferring to eat alone, usually in secret or late at night, to avoid feeling embarrassed.

Contrary to binge eating disorders, adolescents with **bulimia nervosa** would recurrently indulge in the restrictive and/or overeating/purging behaviour mentioned above to compensate for their overeating, and giving too much importance to self-evaluation of their body shape and weight. But children with **binge eating disorders** do feel distressed and may even be guilty after overeating, but they do not excessively compensate for this behaviour.

### How can you identify eating disorders?

As adults working with children, it is important to understand that eating disorders are more complicated than simply unhealthy diets or weight-related issues. The symptoms of eating disorders are a manifestation of underlying emotional issues within children, including poor self-esteem, self-blame, feelings of inferiority, or shame. It is these negative thoughts and feelings that the child is attempting to deal with by using the faulty coping mechanisms of eating disorders.

At times, it can be challenging to determine whether self-conscious adolescents, who are dieting or are concerned about weight, are actually suffering from an eating disorder. Moreover, a person with an eating disorder will often go to great lengths to hide the problem. Astute observation skills, as well as complete and correct information are, therefore, the most necessary tools for you as a front-line professional to ensure the timely identification of the problem.

| Warning Signs of Eating Disorders |
|---|
| • Excessive preoccupation with looks and weight. |
| • Unexplained weight loss/gain. |
| • Excessive physical activity designed to lose weight. |
| • Sudden change in eating habits (food rituals, refusal to eat, sudden change of tastes, etc.). |
| • Avoidance of mealtimes, preferring to eat alone or in secret. |
| • Disappearing after meals, spending excessive time in the bathroom or other secret places. |
| • Hiding high-calorie food or empty food packets in cupboards or drawers. |
| • Food being thrown or emptied in the trash or outside. |
| • Newly developed interest in cooking and food/calories related topics. |
| • Constant comparisons with peers, feeling inferior. |
| • Withdrawal from social gatherings and interactions. |
| • Increase in restlessness and irritability, especially when approaching mealtimes. |

## What causes eating disorders?

Multiple theories and contributing factors have been suggested for the development of eating disorders. There is, however, no consensus on a single causative factor that can be fully implicated. An interaction between genetic, biological, psychosocial as well as cultural factors is believed to be responsible for causing the illness.

*Biological factors:*

Eating disorders involve a disruption in the regulation of the neurotransmitter serotonin, which has also been implicated in depressive and anxiety disorders as well. Additionally, the HPA axis (hypothalamic-pituitary-adrenal axis) also plays a role by regulating hormones that influence eating behaviour and hunger and thirst drives.

*Genetic factors:*

The tendency to develop an eating disorder is also found to run in families. Genetic studies have shown that both anorexia nervosa and bulimia nervosa are heritable disorders. Although eating disorders do occur in males as well, estimates indicate that there are 10 females for every male with an eating disorder.

*Sociocultural factors:*

There is a significant sociocultural component contributing to the development of eating disorders. Peer and media influences play a major role in deciding the idealized body shapes, and the expectations and perceptions related to self-image, especially for children and adolescents, who tend to choose their role models based on perceptions derived from mass media. Furthermore, glamorization and internalization of thin idols, dieting and body dissatisfaction are often ingredients embedded in some cultures.

*Psychological factors:*

Psychological factors like maladaptive attitudes or beliefs about eating, or body shape, identity conflicts, or overvaluation of appearance are associated with eating disorders. Other psychological and social stressors like trauma, childhood abuse, insecure attachment, bullying or dysfunctional families have also been found to contribute to the development of the problem.

## Why is early intervention important?

The high levels of anxiety and denial associated with the illness can make it difficult for a person trying to intervene in the situation. However, it is important to treat a child or teenager affected by the problem with sensitivity while making a special effort to connect with them every day, as eating disorders have the highest mortality rate for any mental illness. Considering that high rate, the earliest possible identification and intervention for such children and adolescents is undeniably necessary, as treatment is most effective if started in the early stages of the disorder. The longer abnormal eating behaviour persists, the more difficult it is to overcome the disorder and its effects on the body. Furthermore, children and adolescents with eating disorders are at risk of harming themselves, as well as for developing other comorbid conditions such as depression, anxiety as well as mood disorders, which makes it increasingly challenging to treat the condition.

For these reasons, **it is imperative to be empowered to prevent such adverse outcomes through ensuring identification at the earliest and provision of adequate and timely psychiatric and psychological intervention.**

## Who is at risk?

Regardless of age, gender, nationality, or culture, any child can be affected by an eating disorder. Furthermore, eating disorders commonly have an onset in childhood as well as adolescence and early adulthood. Different children and adolescents lay different levels of emphasis on their body shapes and eating habits. However, some are more prone to developing unhealthy ways of using food and using unhealthy eating habits as their coping mechanisms.

> ### Red Flags (Beware As These Increase Risk)
> - Anxious, insecure, or perfectionistic disposition.
> - Parent with a history of eating disorder.
> - Difficult and challenging family circumstances.
> - History of childhood abuse—verbal, physical, or sexual.
> - Low sense of self.
> - Low peer group support and other support mechanisms.

## The FSMH steps

### STEP 1: Identify the children at risk

Some behavioural signs that you need to watch out for as an adult working with children include:
- Eating too much or too little.
- Getting irritable and even angry, especially when approaching mealtimes.
- Disappearing to secret hide-outs regularly or right after meals.
- Frequent visits to the bathroom, with running taps to muffle sounds of vomiting.
- Avoiding mealtimes.
- Becoming self-conscious and preoccupied with body image.
- Spending excessive time in front of the mirror or using the weighing scale/measuring tape frequently.
- Constantly making comparisons with peers.
- Suddenly taking interest in cooking, recipes, ingredients and calories.
- Disinterest in being with peers, preferring to be alone.
- Unexplained complaints regarding deterioration of health.
- Lack of attention and concentration.
- Drop in grades and class performance.

## STEP 2: Begin a non-confrontational conversation

- **Don't hesitate to begin the conversation.** As an adult who has identified a child at risk for developing an eating disorder, you could feel hesitant about approaching the subject, fearing a denial due to the child or adolescent's tendency to attempt to hide the symptoms. They are often scared to ask for help, and continue struggling internally within themselves. It is of great value to help such children by talking to them, helping them realize that someone does understand and care about what they are feeling and experiencing.
- **Be non-confrontational.** The few people who might have noticed the child's unhealthy eating patterns might have ticked them off by being critical and blaming them for their wrong habits. Such children and adolescents might experience a low sense of self-esteem and self-worth, at times harbouring the feeling that they do not even deserve to be helped. Active listening and engaging with the child is needed, to be able to express your concerns and demonstrate your support and availability to the child clearly in such a scenario. Avoid being critical, as it could make them defensive as well as defiant.
- **Express your concerns about the child's health without pointing out to the problems with the child.** Even if the child denies the symptoms and refuses to acknowledge their inner conflict, do not get worked up, anxious, or aggressive. Simply communicate your care and concern about their health, at the same time being respectful of their privacy. The child will realize that you are concerned, and might feel comfortable to come back and talk to you at a later time. The existence of such a person to be able to go and talk to, and be understood, can be a major relief for such children.
- **Do not talk about their weight.** Children who may be

displaying symptoms of an eating disorder are usually very self-conscious. Often even an attempt to compliment or praise them does not help in boosting their self-esteem or confidence. Rather, such comments, made with the intention of making them feel better about themselves, could in turn increase their preoccupation with their body image, reinforcing the importance of their weight and shape. You should never say things like 'You're not fat' as such a statement could indicate that being fat is not acceptable.
- **Be reassuring.** Most children and adolescents struggling with such aspects tend to be anxious and insecure, and they need someone to be able to listen to them, empathize and provide reassurance. Do not scare them with the potential consequences of their behaviour in the long-term. Instead, focus on the possibility of seeking help, to overcome the symptoms and work towards a healthier lifestyle.

## STEP 3: Encourage help-seeking and provide information

You can help the child/teenager or their parents feel optimistic and in control of the situation by doing some basic things:

- Provide the reassurance that their experience is a diagnosable and treatable illness.
- Convey that recovery from an eating disorder is possible.
- Reassure them that eating disorders can be adequately treated through psychiatric and psychological interventions.

Eating disorders require adequate medical and psychological intervention. Effective treatment must address both the physical as well as the psychological needs of the child, and hence the role of professional help is irreplaceable, with the goal to fulfil any medical or nutritional needs, promote a healthy relationship with food, and encourage alternative and healthier coping mechanisms.

Often, a combination of therapy, nutritional counselling and support groups works best. In some cases, residential treatment or hospitalization may be necessary, which an expert would be able to guide and help with.

## STEP 4: Talk to parents/caregivers

As a professional working with children, it would be common to be faced with parents or caregivers who would be unaware of what eating disorders are and how they can impact a child. It is vital for you to psychoeducate them to clear the commonly believed myths related to eating disorders and mental health problems, providing them with complete information, while reassuring them about the possible courses of treatment available.

| Busting Myths Related to Eating Disorders |
|---|
| **Eating disorders are a normal part of adolescence**<br>It is important to remember that eating disorder is not a normal phase that adolescents go through with a desire to be thin, and that they will grow out of in time. It is an illness and needs to be treated with medication and therapy. Without treatment, eating disorders can leave a significant impact on the child's health, as they can also be fatal. |
| **Eating disorder is simply a lifestyle choice**<br>Eating disorders are a serious illness with physical and psychological consequences. They are a manifestation of underlying emotional conflicts within the adolescent, and children and adolescents with the illness have maladaptive coping mechanisms. |
| **Recovery from eating disorders is not possible**<br>With early identification, and adequate and timely intervention, an adolescent with an eating disorder can be treated and helped to lead a happier and healthier life. |

## STEP 5: Encourage media literacy as a prevention policy

Advertisements and entertainment media define what is desirable and in vogue, thriving on stereotypical notions of what it means to be attractive and popular. As a prevention strategy for schools as well, it is a must for all children and adolescents to be educated about the media, encouraging them to understand the messages constructed by the media, enhancing their abilities to decipher them and the intent behind their construction. It is essential to bust the misconceptions and misinformation that percolates to them through various media, helping them understand the consequences of their actions and enabling better decision-making. As front-line professionals, you should educate not just children and adolescents about the role of media literacy, but also inform the parents of its priority for today's youth, explaining its impact on eating disorders and body image concerns.

## STEP 6: Build resilience post the intervention

What happens after the child receives treatment is as important as the treatment in itself in any kind of mental health illness. In order to effectively rehabilitate the child, it is important to make his reintegration into society and in his everyday life and routines as smooth as possible. Some things that you need to keep in mind are:

- **Do not overtly treat the child any different from the others**, remember that other children will also take cue from you on how to interact and behave with the child.
- **Educate other children about the illness, its signs, symptoms and effects.** Increase their awareness about the illness and the warning signs associated with it. Try to reduce the stigma by equating mental health illnesses to physical illnesses.

- **Making children aware of the need to process media in a critical manner.** Children frequently do not understand the implications or intent of media messages and it is important that they not consume media without understanding or evaluating these messages completely.
- **Express hope and optimism to motivate the child** towards resuming a healthy lifestyle, and encourage his efforts towards the same.
- **Help the child explore his talents to boost his self-confidence** and to shift the preoccupation from body image to more achievement-oriented tasks.
- **Talk about body image and its related aspects.** For the child it is important that there is a balance in his views about his body and his own self which would make it imperative that there be an understanding of the need for a healthy body and not necessarily a thin one.
- **Help the child realize that there is more to defining what is good and what is not in an individual.** It is imperative that the child learns to evaluate himself in the context of his abilities and skills, and not in terms of how he looks.
- **Work on helping the child build good relationships** with friends and family.
- **Help the child build more effective coping mechanisms** by working on problem-solving through various brainstorming exercises and making them see solutions in problems where they do not see any.
- **Help the child develop better thinking skills.** It is going to be essential for the child with a history of eating disorders to be able to think through situations carefully and comprehensively and you would play an important role in helping the child develop the right skills for that.
- **Maintain contact with the parents and if possible with the treating mental health professional** to ensure that regular

and consistent follow-ups are being done with regard to the illness.

Changes in appetite and eating patterns can appear to be normal. However, to the discerning eye these changes can indicate the development of an eating disorder. The challenge lies in breaking through the strong identification that the child or adolescent may have with maintaining a certain body type and building acceptance towards the problem.

# 14

# SUBSTANCE USE DISORDERS

Alcohol and drug addiction is a common challenge among adolescents that has a far-reaching negative impact on their physical, emotional and psychological development. Addiction can be understood as the continued use of mood-altering substances despite detrimental effects on the body, mind and the immediate surroundings of the individual.

The teen years are a critical period of development, and adolescents are given to be experimental with much risk taking behaviour including the use and abuse of drugs and alcohol. The line between casual use and drug abuse is thin and dangerous, and more often than not, addiction sneaks up on the adolescent with a gradual increase in use as it begins to fulfil a valuable need in the eyes of the user—this need could be anything from mood elevation to pain relief. Some teenagers may turn to substances simply out of curiosity or even as a faulty coping mechanism to deal with their feelings of loneliness, depression, stress, anxiety, or to cope with family-related problems and stressors.

## Understanding substance abuse

Substance abuse can take place in many forms—prescription drugs are usually taken orally, while other drugs can be smoked, inhaled or taken intravenously. Drugs commonly fall under the following categories.

- Narcotics (heroin and morphine)
- Stimulants (cocaine, nicotine)
- Depressants (alcohol, sedatives)
- Cannabis (marijuana and hashish)
- Hallucinogens (LSD, ecstasy)
- Inhalants (glue, paint products, diluter)
- Steroids

Substance abuse is not the occasional use of alcohol or other substances. It involves continued and frequent use of substances, despite being aware of its negative consequences to the person's functioning at familial, academic and social levels over a period of time. Substance dependence occurs when the adolescent consuming it has become more tolerant of the substance, meaning that he needs to consume more of the substance than was previously required, in order to achieve the same level of 'high'. Adolescents who have developed a dependency on a substance would not be able to give it up without experiencing withdrawals, which are the immediate effects of discontinuing a substance after prolonged use.

To qualify as a **substance use disorder**, the following aspects need to be present:

- **Dependence on the substance**. The drug use goes out of the control of the user and he will continue using it even if he means not to and wants to stop. Substance abuse will have replaced other activities and relationships.
- **Disrupting daily life of the person**. The adolescent is unable to carry on leading a normal life because of his drug use. Risk-taking behaviour like reckless driving, increased aggression, and unprotected sex become common and the adolescent totally ignores daily responsibilities due to the substance use as he is preoccupied with procuring the drug for use, thereby hampering his physical, social as well as

educational functioning.
- **Evident mental and physical health consequences**. Despite the awareness that drug use is hurting them, as it may be causing blackouts, memory loss, infection, depression, psychosis, to name a few, the adolescent would still continue to use it.

## Facts

- According to the National Institute of Drug Abuse (2004), an estimated 22.5 million persons over the age of 12 were classified as suffering from substance related disorders.
- Men are much more likely than women to be binge drinkers and heavy drinkers (Saddock, Saddock & Ruiz, 2015).

## Signs and symptoms of substance abuse

The typical symptoms which are seen when a child/adolescent has become habituated to using a drug and when there is dependence on the same include the following:

- **Physical, behavioural and psychological withdrawal symptoms**. Attempts to stop the usage of substances can lead to the experiencing of withdrawal symptoms which could include sweating, tremors, nausea, or sleeplessness. The user in this case would continue to use the substance in order to prevent the onset of the withdrawal symptoms.
- The **adolescent's tolerance level goes up** and he needs more and more of the substance to feel the 'hit'. This happens as the adolescent's reaction, to the same quantity of the substance gets reduced over a period of prolonged use, thereby making him progressively increase the quantity of consumption. Such a tolerance could be both physiological as well as psychological, leading to increased cravings for the substance in use.

- All of the adolescent's time is spent **preoccupied with either procuring the substance or using it**. Due to this, there is a significant reduction in other adaptive and occupational activities
- There is a significant **loss of control** and the adolescent feels compelled to use the substance 'despite himself' and the negative consequences of consuming it.
- There are typically two patterns relating to misusing substances. Either the adolescent has become a regular user in which case he or she will need to use the substance every day and possibly several times a day. On the other hand, the adolescent might be a binger in which case he may not take drugs or drink alcohol for some time (usually a few days) and then will binge or take many drugs or large quantities of alcohol at once.

## How can you identify substance abuse?

As an individual working closely with children and adolescents, it is essential that you have an understanding of some of the aspects of substance use and its abuse that would allow you to be able to identify the problem at the earliest. It is important to remember that it is the presence of multiple aspects or areas of concern as well as the continuity of their existence over a period of time which tends to indicate towards the existence of a problem. No single sign in itself can be treated as an indicant of the problem.

| Warning Signs of Susbtance Abuse |
| --- |
| • Red glazed eyes |
| • Excessive fatigue |
| • Increased irritability |
| • Temperamental behaviour |

| |
|---|
| • Isolating self |
| • Sudden academic decline |
| • Lack of interest in activities |
| • Poor judgement in situations |
| • Increased impulsivity |
| • Money disappearing from home |

## What causes substance use disorders?

Numerous factors have been linked to the development of the problem of drug use and their abuse. Often the precipitation of the problem is a result of the presence of multiple factors and not a singular factor.

*Neurobiological factors:*

An important neurological substrate that mediates drug abuse is the midbrain dopamine system, which represents the reward system of the brain. Drugs activate the reward system to increase dopamine release, thereby enhancing the pleasure pathways of the brain with repeated administration. Moreover, repeated use of drugs may lead to lessening of prefrontal 'reflective' processes and a corresponding increase in striatal activity which underpins habitual behaviour.

*Genetic factors:*

Genetic factors may contribute to the problem of drug abuse, although studies remain inconclusive. A genetic predisposition or biological vulnerability is not sufficient, and the role of environmental factors cannot be discounted. At best, drug abuse, like any other clinical disorder, may be best explained by gene-environment interaction.

*Psychosocial factors:*

Disrupted families with parents who abuse drugs may underlie learning behaviour of drug abuse in children. Difficulties in stress tolerance and negative affectivity like anxiety and somatic complaints have also been correlated with repeated drug abuse. Difficulties in interpersonal relationships and conflicts have also been found to be contributing factors.

*Personal factors:*

Drug users who develop problems have personal vulnerability before they begin taking drugs. Associated behaviour like truancy, delinquency and poor school record have been observed. Traits such as aggressiveness, sensation seeking and impulsivity are also common. Studies have also focused on links between drug abuse and other clinical disorders like depression, schizophrenia and antisocial personality.

*Social environment related factors:*

Drug abuse is influenced by peers or parents. Within the immediate group, there might be social pressure to take drugs to achieve status. Studies have also found a link between drug misuse and indices of social deprivation, such as unemployment and homelessness. The easy availability of drugs (either legally by prescription or from illicit sources) is an important factor in drug abuse.

## Why is early intervention important?

Regardless of the nature of the substance that is being abused, addiction causes significant changes in the brain that further perpetuates the addiction cycle. Drug use causes a rise in dopamine levels, making the experience pleasurable along with giving rise to a consequent desire to repeat this pleasurable event. In addictions, using the drug is given the same importance as survival behaviour such as fulfilling hunger or thirst. The physiological and psychological changes in the brain and body lead to clouding of judgement and thought clarity, making it difficult for the adolescent to function normally without the drug. The level of insight among those who abuse substances is very poor and they typically find many rationalizations to justify their drug use and the level of control they have over its consumption. An addiction is rather difficult to treat, especially when it has been present for a long time. There is no substitute for early intervention when it comes to drug abuse as it has serious negative consequences for the individual's health, their social relationships, academic and occupational life.

### Who is at risk?

While an adolescent abusing a substance cannot inevitably be blamed to be a victim of circumstances, it is important to note that certain factors may make a child more susceptible to developing a substance use disorder. Having a knowledge of these factors is imperative to ensure that you can identify these problems at the earliest and take a proactive approach to taking care of them.

---

**Red Flags (Beware As These Increase Risk)**

- Exposure to substance use in significant family members.
- Significant traumatic life event such as abuse or neglect.
- Early exposure to substances in peer group.
- Previous mental health conditions like depression or psychosis.
- Low self-esteem.
- Aggressive or disruptive tendencies.

## The FSMH steps

### STEP 1: Identify the child at risk

If you notice the physical, social, or emotional signs of a suspected addiction problem, it is important for you to explore this possibility further. These signs have been discussed above and are enlisted in detail below. As adults working with children, it is not only important for you to be on the lookout for such warning signs, but also talk about them openly, to encourage children to share and report the same.

1. *Physical signs*

- Fatigue
- Repeated health complaints
- Red glazed eyes
- Lasting cough

2. *Emotional changes*

- Personality change
- Sudden mood changes
- Irritability
- Irresponsible behaviour
- Low self-esteem
- Poor judgement
- Depression
- General lack of interest
- Temper tantrums

3. *Social changes*

- Sudden jitteriness or nervousness
- Increased secretiveness
- Continual wearing of long-sleeved clothes and sunglasses to hide the telltale signs of injection marks or redness of eyes

- Withdrawal and social isolation
- Deterioration in physical appearance and grooming
- Association with known substance abusers
- Unusual borrowing of money

4. *Changes in relation to family*

- Breaking of rules
- Frequent arguments
- Withdrawing from family
- Unusual borrowing of money
- Stealing small items
- Secretive behaviour
- Escaping from responsibilities

5. *Changes at school*

- Loss of interest
- Negative attitude
- Deterioration in results
- Absenteeism
- Truancy
- Discipline problems
- Frequent trips to the restroom

## STEP 2: Assess for risky behaviour

Prior to intervening, it is necessary to assess the risk associated with the child or adolescent's behaviour associated with consumption of a substance. Its use can significantly alter an adolescent's thinking, perception and judgement, thereby increasing the likelihood of risk-taking or reckless behaviour. If a person is an addict, you need to be aware of the fact that he can also be in danger of harming self or others. You will need to assess the risk of such a behaviour that a person can engage in. Some aspects relating to this are discussed in the chapter pertaining to suicide and self-harm.

## STEP 3: Listen and reassure

Alcohol and drug abuse can bring about an immense feeling of loss of control, guilt, helplessness and hopelessness. Typically children and adolescents tend to deny the presence of a problem which can be difficult to break. There is significant stigma in the society which means that the adolescent might find it very difficult to share their concerns with another person. In order to be truly empathic, you need to be aware of your own biases regarding drug and alcohol use.

You will need to listen to the individual non-judgementally and without criticism. It is important to not vent out frustration to the conversation. It is important that you do not scold or patronize the adolescent. If they are expressing their fears and anxieties to you, it is important that you really listen. Appreciate the courage that it would take for them to share their innermost feelings and fears with you. In a non-threatening manner, try and explore the extent and nature of the substance use and reassure the adolescent about the possibility of intervention. It is essential to instil hope and support in the child to enable future work and recovery.

## STEP 4: Inform the parent/caregiver

In cases of an addiction, not just the adolescent but the whole family also becomes part of the cycle and suffers equally. As a professional working with children and adolescents, you might be faced with an adolescent whom you have identified as abusing a substance, but the adolescent refuses to take your help or where the family is unaware of the existence of a problem. In such situations, it is vital for you to first inform the parent or caregiver.

Remember to communicate with the parents in a clear but empathic manner, informing them that addiction is a real medical condition and would require treatment. While the child/adolescent is not a victim of circumstances, it is important for the caregivers to be aware that some adolescents are more prone to suffer from addiction problems, and environmental stressors can be significant contributors to it. They need to be reassured and provided with a comprehensive understanding of the treatment options available to them for helping their child and also remember to be patient and answer all their questions.

### Busting Myths About Substance Abuse

**Using and abusing substances is a voluntary behaviour**
Substance abuse is a complex neurological disorder that is formed due to multiple interactions between biological, social, family and genetic factors. While the adolescent may voluntarily decide to experiment with drugs initially, however, as time passes the person becomes a compulsive user and the drug takes control over his behaviour and motivations. Continued drug use causes changes in the brain that begin to treat the drug as important for survival behaviour.

**Addiction to substances is a character flaw**
Addiction is an illness and must be viewed as such. Every drug affects the brain's functioning in its own unique way. What all drug users have in common, however, is that drug use becomes the single most important motivator over time. This is because the drug alters the person's behaviour, thought and actions in fundamental ways. You cannot be free of addiction simply through willpower. It is a medical illness.

| **Addiction cannot be treated** |
|---|
| It is extremely difficult for people addicted to drugs to achieve and maintain long-term abstinence. However, with the help of professional support it is possible to be rid of this problem. For adolescents in particular it is important to intervene and stop substance abuse as early as possible, as children become addicted to drugs much faster than adults and are at a higher risk for physical, mental and psychological harm from illicit drug use if it remains untreated. |
| **Treatment for drug addiction is not long-term and intensive** |
| In most cases, treatment for drug addiction is long-term, at multiple levels, and often repeated. This is because drug addiction is a chronic disease and each individual will have unique issues related to his drug use that need to be taken care of in a specific and individualized manner. |

## STEP 5: Encourage help-seeking and provide information

It is important for you to direct the child or adolescent's parents to seek the help of professional experts including psychiatrists and psychologists who are trained to deal with such problems with the help of medications as well as psychotherapy for their child. Parents can have significant reservations in meeting with mental health professionals and it would be important that you take care of these concerns by helping them understand that this is a medical illness like any other and needs to be treated. In the case of substance use and its abuse, there is no substitute for intervention by professionals. Support and motivation are a very important part of a successful recovery from addiction, and once a person has developed a dependence on a substance, there is a significant risk of relapse. Counselling in such a scenario for the recovering individual as well as the family is of utmost importance.

## STEP 6: Building resilience post the intervention

Since relapse is a real ever-present danger, it is important to encourage the development and maintenance of self-help strategies in the adolescents. Following are some of the things that you can look at in order to ensure that the individual is able to cope effectively and stays away from substances in the future:

- **Involve family and friends** to ensure that they have an adequate support structure.
- **Encourage social-skills training** for them because it has often been observed that children who abuse drugs tend to have deficits in dealing with social situations.
- **Establish a system of pro-social peers** who could promote the reporting and sharing of such behaviour, can make themselves available to talk to the individual when needed if they have a craving, and would also help the individual stay away from substances.
- **Ensure the development of a drug-free environment in school or the community** by having awareness programmes.
- **Encourage children to talk about their experiences** to ensure that there is no stigma that develops around the problem the child has gone through.
- **Equip them with life-skills such as assertiveness,** to deal with difficult social situations and to be able to say no to peer pressure or any other such difficult situation.
- **Enable students to make more effective choices** by brain storming around challenging situations that can arise and how to solve them in an efficacious manner.

## STEP 7: Work towards designing ways of preventing substance abuse

As a front-line professional, it is important that you also look at ways in which you could ensure the prevention of the development of a problem like substance abuse. It is important to talk about and discuss the problem of drugs in the school or community where you work in. Sharing experiences and encouraging students to talk while also implementing strategies such as encouraging adolescents to learn to say 'NO' (being assertive) to avoid succumbing to pressure from peers and others are some ways forward. Social-skills and assertiveness training can be encouraged as major tools to empower the youth to protect themselves from falling prey to substance abuse. An open communication system should be developed, to ensure that the children can build a rapport with you, and can trust you to share their feelings and thoughts. Such a policy would also help the adolescents understand the need for seeking help. At the same time, it is essential to have clear reporting systems in place such that the child or adolescent knows where he needs to go in case there is a problem, who is the right person to contact, and how the contact needs to be made.

# 15
# SCHIZOPHRENIA IN CHILDREN AND ADOLESCENTS

Schizophrenia has been a much talked about illness, both in media and otherwise. Most individuals have their own understandings and connotations attached to it. For many, it is typically associated with what is traditionally considered to be insanity or madness since numerous misconceptions remain associated with it. There is immense fear, stigma and shame that move hand-in-hand with schizophrenia and people more often than not refrain from talking about its symptoms and manifestations on account of how they would be viewed by others. As a result, there is a significant challenge in encouraging help-seeking by patients and their families and in creating an environment of openness for discussion about its signs and symptoms to promote early intervention and treatment.

Schizophrenia in children manifests itself in a similar way to that in adults with disruptive psychopathology emerging in their cognition, emotion, perception and behaviour. However, a significant challenge emerges in the ability to distinguish and differentiate it from childhood experiences which may be normal—such as creative play which may include imaginary characters and self-talk.

Thus, it is essential that you, in your work as a teacher, counsellor, parent or social worker, are equipped with the right information, the knowledge of symptoms and risk factors as well as support and intervention methods to take care of the child and the problem in an efficacious manner.

## Facts

- Studies have reported lifetime prevalence rates for schizophrenia at 1.1 per cent worldwide. Prevalence rate of schizophrenia in India is estimated to be 4.3–8.7 million (Regier, Narrow, Rae, Manderscheid, Locke & Goodwin, 1993).
- Childhood-onset schizophrenia occurs in less than one out of 10,000 children (Saddock, Saddock & Ruiz, 2015).
- Prevalence rates of schizophrenia in adolescents are 50 times higher than in children, estimated at 1–2 per 1000 (Saddock, Saddock & Ruiz, 2015).
- Suicide is the leading cause of premature death and these attempts are made by 20–50 per cent of the patients. This is 20 times more than that in the general population (Saddock, Saddock & Ruiz, 2015).

## Signs and symptoms of schizophrenia

Schizophrenia refers to a group of illnesses with varied presentations, bringing with it negative implications in all domains of functioning of the individual. Often in the case of children, the symptoms do not present in a florid manner immediately. Rather they tend to develop and grow slowly over a period of time, and initially may be represented only in the form of oddities in speech and behaviour.

The typical symptoms which are observed in schizophrenia include the following:

- Children may frequently hear voices commenting on their actions or commanding them to do things which are called

- **auditory hallucinations**.
- They may also see giants, monsters and scary creatures, experiencing them as real stimuli in the outside environment (**visual hallucinations**) which can be an extremely frightening experience for the child.
- They can develop false beliefs about themselves, others and the world which are held with strong conviction (**delusions**). For example, the child may believe that people are looking at him and are trying to harm him in some way. Often such beliefs are accompanied by acting out against them such as being very cautious and suspicious of people, not leaving the house due to the fear of one's safety, to name a few.
- Thoughts may be affected and thinking may become illogical. This is manifest in speech, as a result of which speech would lack meaningful content and communication may be used only to convey basic needs.
- Many behavioural symptoms such as inappropriate smiling, giggling or crying may be present. Children may be aggressive and have anger outbursts.
- They may not show much concern for their health and hygiene.

## How can you identify schizophrenia?

Besides the prominent signs and symptoms which can indicate towards the presence or the onset of the condition, there are some other subtle aspects which can act as warning signs suggestive of a problem. In your work with children and adolescents, it may not always be easy to identify the prominent symptoms as the illness has an insidious onset, which means that it develops in a slow and gradual manner. Some aspects which you should keep in mind include the following:

- Children with the disorder may show significant developmental abnormalities prior to the onset of the disorder.

- There may be disinterest in activities that keep other children engaged such as school, social interactions and play.
- They would display limited social skills and tend to be clingy and may not be responsive to social cues and situations.
- It may be difficult to motivate a child with the problem to engage in any kind of activity against their wish.
- Their patterns of responding may appear odd and idiosyncratic, making it difficult to understand the reasoning behind their actions.
- Inappropriate emotional responses may be seen with a difficulty to express as much as other children would normally be able to.

| Warning Signs of Schizophrenia |
|---|
| • Appearing withdrawn and lost in thoughts. |
| • Illogical reasoning or explanations for problems. |
| • Feeling persecuted or that people will cause harm. |
| • Being distrustful of peers and adults. |
| • Engaging in excessive talking to self. |
| • Poor judgement, decision-making and problem-solving. |
| • Excessive aggression and hostility. |
| • Inappropriate emotional responses to social situations. |

## What causes schizophrenia?

Schizophrenia has multiple contributing factors which in conjunction with each other lead to the precipitation of the disorder. These include genetic, biological and psychosocial aspects.

*Genetic factors:*

Heritability has been understood as being the most important factor in childhood-onset schizophrenia. It has been found that it is eight times more prevalent in immediate family members of a child diagnosed with the illness than in the general population. Chromosome linkages have also been implicated in the transmission of the illness, though the exact mechanism of heredity is not completely understood.

### Biological factors:

Neurological abnormalities such as impairments in sustaining attention, processing information, intelligence and memory have been found in children suffering from the illness. Loss of cell volume in certain areas of the brain has also been found. Dysregulation of chemicals in the brain called neurotransmitters (primarily Dopamine) has been associated and provides rationale for treatment with medication that alters neurotransmitter regulation. Other risk factors associated with schizophrenia include age above 50 years of the father at conception of the child, exposure to toxins during pregnancy of the mother and complications at the time of birth.

### Psychosocial factors:

Biological vulnerability interacts with environmental stressors to manifest as symptoms. Neglectful or overly critical parenting, poor relatedness with family members, unstable home environments, high levels of expressed emotions (negative interactions characterized by hostility, criticalness and over-involvement) by family members, conflicting and contradictory messages and other stressors have been associated with the onset and relapse of the illness.

## Why is early intervention important?

The challenge posited by schizophrenia with an onset in childhood, is the poor prognosis which is associated with the illness. The earlier the onset of the illness, the more difficult it can be to treat it, with higher chances of relapses and recurrences in the future as well. An early identification in the case of schizophrenia is exceptionally important given the impact it can have upon the whole life of the individual, compromising the ability to recover fully from it, which also increases the risk for self-harm.

**Early identification by being more aware of the early signs and risk factors can prevent the full onset of the illness, thus, providing better chances for the child to lead a normal life in the future, unaffected by the negative aspects of having had the illness at an early age.**

## Who is at risk?

Like any illness, the presence of some factors or aspects can increase the risk of having schizophrenia at an early age as well.

### Red Flags (Beware As These Increase Risk)

- Family history of schizophrenia.
- Exposure to viruses, toxins, or malnutrition while in the womb or perinatal trauma.
- History of neurological signs and symptoms.
- Older age of the father at the time of conception.
- Early developmental abnormalities—delayed milestones.
- Taking psychoactive drugs during teen years.
- Very few friends, preferring to be alone.
- History of aggression or assault.
- Bizarre experiences—feeling of being out of one's body, etc.

## The FSMH steps

### STEP 1: Identify the early signs and symptoms in children

Awareness of changes in behaviour and thinking may lead to early intervention. Besides the aspects discussed previously in the chapter, these changes may manifest as:

- Disturbance in sleep
- Aggression and anger outbursts
- Odd behaviour—talking to oneself, smiling to oneself
- Suspiciousness and fearfulness
- Use of drugs and other substances
- Lack of concentration or an inability to make simple decisions
- Decline in academic performance

### STEP 2: Assess the stressors and rule out other possible reasons for the signs

It is important to understand the onset of the symptoms and whether they were triggered by any stressor other than schizophrenia. If a child has symptoms they must be understood in the light of the current situations in the child's life and also must be distinguished from other disorders of mood and anxiety or any other problem. In case of schizophrenia in a child, the behaviour is likely to appear strange and he may not be able to verbalize any structured thoughts of hopelessness or of suicide or anxiety. His fears may be vague and diffuse and he may not be able to explain them. **You need to be absolutely certain that there is a significant problem before you go on to the next step as you would not want to create unnecessary panic.**

## STEP 3: Involve the family and share your concern with them

As someone working closely with the child, you would have observed some signs and symptoms which may be worrisome and cause you to think that a significant problem like schizophrenia may be precipitating. It would be imperative to corroborate the same with the family to ensure that what is happening is not specific to one context and is the overall experience of the child's life as reflected at school, home and in the community with peers and relatives.

Making the family aware of the child's symptoms is essential as any help-seeking cannot be initiated without the family's consent. Providing the parents/caregivers with necessary information and emphasizing on the need for early intervention is essential. There are some aspects which should be kept in mind while talking to the families and breaking the news of the problem to them.

### Breaking the news to parents:

- There is significant fear, anxiety, shame, stigma and misconceptions that are associated with an illness like schizophrenia. This would imply that you need to **be extremely sensitive, slow, calm and focused in your communication with parents.**
- **Do not use jargon and talk to the families in easily understandable language** which is comprehensible for them, helping them connect with what you are observing so that you can get them on board with the fact that there is a problem which needs to be addressed.
- **Anticipate a panic reaction from the family.** This would ensure that you are better prepared to handle them, their response and the situation, ensuring that they move forward

in the right direction.
- **Give the family a comprehensive understanding of what to expect, what the illness is and how they can help the child in overcoming the situation.** Share information and literature and encourage them to talk to experts to enhance their understanding of the problem.
- **Remind them to not blame the child.** Ensure that they understand this is a medical problem which needs to be treated as such and is not something that the child is doing to himself. It is important for the family to understand that there is nothing that the child could have done to prevent the problem.
- Help the family understand that even though there are factors which can increase the risk of having the disorder which relate to the family, **blaming their own selves cannot take away from the biological underpinnings of the problem.** It is essential to emphasize that instead of finding people or things to blame it would be important to instead shift to a problem-solving mode to take care of the condition.

## STEP 4: Encourage help-seeking in parents

As the individual working closely with children and adolescents, it would be your role to create a bridge between the caregivers and the doctor. It would be imperative to ensure that the parent does seek medical intervention from a psychiatrist, as that would form the cornerstone of the treatment in case of schizophrenia. Early intervention during the initial stages of the illness needs to involve medications and psychosocial support to improve symptoms and delay or prevent progression to the full-blown illness.

It is equally important to handle the caregivers' reactions with empathy and reflective listening as once they have started seeking treatment they may be struck by the enormity of the condition and would require support. Their myths and fears about the illness need to be clarified patiently. They must be educated about their role in caregiving. Changes in communication patterns in the family must be emphasized, so as to reduce critical reactions and stressful interactions. The family members must be trained to reward small positive changes in the patient's behaviour. The importance of family involvement in preventing a relapse must be stressed upon.

| Busting Myths Related to Schizophrenia |
|---|
| **Schizophrenia is not an illness that is treatable** <br> It is important to remember that schizophrenia is an illness and needs to be treated with medication primarily and therapy conjointly. Without treatment, it can leave a significant impact on the child's health. |
| **Isolating the child is going to be helpful** <br> Early misconceptions of isolating and shunning the individual displaying the symptoms of the illness need to be dispelled. Not isolation but medication and reintegration into normal life is the solution and the way forward. |
| **The child is the cause for the illness** <br> The illness precipitates due to imbalances in the levels of neurotransmitters in the brain and it is not because the child does or does not do something that has resulted in the disorder. Blaming the child in such a scenario only worsens the symptoms and impacts him negatively, affecting both recovery and prognosis. |

You must be prepared to work individually with the caregivers to lessen their burden and prevent a burnout. Be approachable to family members while maintaining boundaries and provide avenues for ventilation and supportive counselling.

## Continuing communication with the family:

- **Listen attentively** and allow the person to express himself freely.

- Provide a safe and **non- judgemental** environment for them.
- Express **validation** and understanding of the family's struggles and fears.
- **Reflect** their feelings and thoughts to make them feel understood as well as to make them aware of their own emotions.
- Help consolidate their thoughts and feelings which they may find very overwhelming by **summarizing** for them.
- **Reduce blame** on self and help them see the biological aspects of the illness.
- **Reassure** the caregiver in a realistic manner creating optimism and hope for the future.
- Help the caregiver **share the burden** of care with other family members or friends.
- **Encourage development of interests and continued pursuit of vocational and professional goals** in the caregiver so that he can feel a sense of purpose and success in his own endeavours.

## STEP 5: Reintegration and rehabilitation

An important step is to assess what the child is capable of doing after the onset of the illness and after seeing his response to treatment. Then a concrete plan for the future must be prepared involving the family and the school/agency.

### Overall aspects of rehabilitation to be focused on:

- **Reintegration into the previous setting** would be ideal.
- Options to **complete education through less intense means** like open school or distance learning should be considered if in case regular schooling would be difficult.
- **Vocational training which means training in specific skills aimed at employment must be initiated,** particularly if

it is felt that education may get compromised due to the debilitating effects of the illness. The skills must be chosen keeping in mind the child's interests and likelihood of those skills yielding employment.
- **Work on reducing cognitive deficits** and specifically training in attention enhancement and memory tasks as well by the use of small activities.
- **Social skills should be worked on in a hierarchical and sequential manner.** It should start with the enhancing the child's ability to understand emotions, moving to expressing feelings with the family, learning effective coping skills, enhancing skills at socialization with people outside of family and finally generalizing to other situations.

## Steps to be taken in the school/community where you are to facilitate reintegration:

- **Ensure that a sense of understanding is built in other members** to ensure there is no ridiculing, blaming, teasing, or bullying.
- **Encourage other children and adults to have positive interactions** with the child who is being reintegrated into the set-up.
- **Create an environment that welcomes the child back by making other individuals more sensitized to his needs** which would include being slow in placing demands relating to work, allowing the child space and time to rebuild relationships and reducing expectations in terms of overall performance.
- **Provide the child multiple opportunities** to be able to determine what activities he would be most comfortable in pursuing.
- **Accommodations may need to be made in terms of changing the goals and academic milestones** that need

to be achieved as per curriculum.
- **Reassure the child of your presence so he can seek help and share anything which happens during the day with you.** Actively work with the child to handle challenging situations that may get highlighted in interactions with him while being gentle and nurturing in your approach.

Schizophrenia remains associated with fear and misconceptions, making diagnosis and treatment a challenging process. Its earliest identification is instrumental in working towards ensuring an early resolution to the illness. Working on the symptoms of the illness, rehabilitation and reintegration are the right steps forward.

# 16
# INTELLECTUAL DISABILITY

There are times when we come across some children who may not look or act their age, and do not seem to be as bright or as able to do things as other children their age. We cannot help but wonder what could have gone wrong, and often make judgements about all the factors that could be influencing the child, including the family, the schooling, the peers, or even the community.

## Understanding intellectual disability

The term **intellectual disability**, (earlier referred to as mental retardation), describes an aspect which is characterized by a below average mental capacity and skills necessary for carrying out functions of day-to-day living. It leads to limitations in the child's intellectual functioning (as reflected in the Intelligence Quotient), that is, his ability for learning, reasoning, decision-making and problem-solving as well as in basic adaptive skills like effective communication, social interaction, self-care, to name a few.

## Facts

- Intellectual disability is believed to affect 2 per cent of the population (NIMH, 2000).

- In India it is estimated that about 20 million people fall in the category of mild mental retardation, and about 4 million people in moderate and severe level of retardation (NIMH, 2000).
- The highest incidence is in school-age children, with the peak at ages 10 to 14 years, being 1.5 times more common in males than among females (Saddock, Saddock & Ruiz, 2015).

## Signs and symptoms of intellectual disability

One of the major signs of an intellectual disability is a global delay in the attainment of various developmental milestones, including the age at which the child is able to roll over, crawl, walk and speak, which can be ascertained by obtaining a history from the child's parents/caregivers. While each child may attain these milestones at their own pace, an approximate check needs to be maintained, as an overall delayed development is strongly suggestive of an intellectual disability. Besides this, intellectual disability in children can be seen in different forms from infancy to adulthood, depending on the level of severity.

### During infancy and childhood

- Delayed or inappropriate sensory response to environmental stimulation.
- Delayed motor skills development.
- Deficits in communication skills including speech and language.
- Inappropriate social and emotional response.
- Frequent behavioural problems like tantrums.
- Inability to apply basic functional academic skills in daily activities.

### During adolescence and adulthood

- Loss of coping and skills related to self-care.

- Significantly below average scholastic performance.
- Difficulty in appropriate reasoning and judgement about environmental events.
- Inability to connect actions with consequences.
- Very few friends and lack of social skills.
- Difficulty in performing vocational and social roles and responsibilities.

Other problems like seizures, motor handicaps, or problems with vision or hearing may also be present in children with a severe or profound intellectual disability.

## How can you identify intellectual disability?

As an adult working with children and adolescents you would be interacting with children presenting with varying levels of learning skills as well as performances. But every child who might be lagging behind his peer need not necessarily be intellectually disabled. Therefore, it is important for you to be aware of the ways in which such children's behaviour can be identified.

| Behavioural Manifestations of Intellectual Disability |
| --- |
| • Lack of friends |
| • Peer rejection or isolation |
| • Preferring to interact with children of a younger age group |
| • Difficulty in taking care of self as is appropriate to age |
| • Lagging behind peers in academics |
| • Frequent behavioural complaints by teachers/parents |
| • Appears to be a slow learner |
| • Displays difficulty in understanding rules |
| • Failure to avoid risky situations |
| • Lack of curiosity |

It is essential to also remember that in order to identify someone as having an intellectual disability it needs to be based on impairments in the child's adaptive functioning, rather than a deficit in intelligence itself. You and the caregivers—together need to evaluate the child's coping skills with daily life demands as expected of children in the similar age ranges. On the other hand, the level of intellectual functioning needs to be ascertained through the use of standardized measures of intelligence tests by mental health professionals trained to do so.

## What causes intellectual disability?

While a large number of cases of intellectual disability usually have unidentified aetiologies, research has evidenced a number of factors which can contribute to the development of an intellectual disability in a child.

### Genetic factors:

Intellectual disability has been strongly indicated to be heritable, as it could be a result of abnormal genes inherited from the biological parents or complexities in gene combination.

### Birth and delivery related conditions:

a) *Prenatal conditions:*

There are many factors related to the mother during pregnancy that could adversely influence the child's development since the time of conception itself. Factors such as maternal diseases, physical infections, stress, alcohol/drug use by the pregnant mother, exposure to radiation, and lack of proper nutritional care during delivery can interfere with the normal development of the fetus and may result in the development of an intellectual disability in the child.

b) *Perinatal conditions:*

Intellectual disability can also result through problems during labour and birthing, like lack of respiration, head trauma, abnormal positioning, premature birth or low birth weight— all of which might have an adverse impact on the development of the child.

c) *Postnatal conditions:*

The period immediately after the birth of the child is also extremely crucial, as health problems like extreme malnutrition, inappropriate medical care, exposure to chemicals, severe jaundice or any head injury may also increase the chances of the development of an intellectual disability.

*Environmental factors:*

The environment can play a role in contributing to the aetiology of an intellectual disability, as lack of adequate physical and mental stimulation in the environment necessary for a child's development could impair the child's learning abilities. Family instability, frequent moves, and multiple but inadequate caregivers may deprive a child of necessary nurturance, leading to a potential risk to the developing brain. Moreover, children who have endured such adverse environmental conditions like poverty and malnutrition have been found to be subject to long-lasting damage to their physical as well as emotional development.

**Why is early identification important?**

The significance of the earliest identification of an intellectual disability cannot be emphasized enough, as the warning signs can actually be identified since infancy itself. Furthermore, the sooner such a child is identified, the greater are the chances for a more successful intervention and the development of compensatory skills.

Children with an intellectual disability are able to learn and perform new skills, but they develop them at a slower rate, taking longer to inculcate and perform basic activities than expected of other children in the same age range if they are provided adequate support, guidance, training and rehabilitation. However, this is not to say that all deficits can be compensated for always.

Furthermore, intellectually disabled children usually lack an appropriate judgement, and thereby are often incapable of ensuring their personal safety. Such children become more prone to facing taunts and rejections, and in the need for approval and friendship, they tend to become highly suggestible. This increases their vulnerability to be at risk for being victims of abuse and other forms of exploitations.[9]

## Who is at risk?

Some children are more prone to develop intellectual disability, and there are certain factors that have been identified to implicate a higher risk for such children or adolescents.

| Red Flags (Beware As These Increase Risk) |
| --- |
| • Complications in pregnancy
• Exposure to toxic substances before or during infancy
• Head injury or other early traumatic experiences
• Environmental deprivation in childhood
• Family history of an intellectual disability |

---

[9]The topic of Trauma and Abuse is discussed in more detail in chapter 19.

## The FSMH steps

### STEP 1: Identify the children at risk

As has been emphasized above, an early identification is the first step to take towards providing help for an intellectually disabled child. It is important for you to be on the lookout for the warning signs mentioned previously, observing the child's behaviour and assessing his level of adaptive functioning in various domains. This would also require gathering information from diverse sources including the parents or caregivers, the school and community in which the child engages and spends time.

### STEP 2: Talk to parents/caregivers

It is of utmost importance to talk to the parents and caregivers as soon as the possibility of an intellectual disability is suspected. Providing parents or guardians with the required information about the illness and the need for early intervention is a must as this is the only method of ensuring the right kind of help is provided to the child.

- **Be prepared for denial.** It would not be uncommon for you to be faced with parents in denial, as no parent would like to acknowledge a problem with their child. It can be an anxiety-provoking situation for the parent, especially when an intellectual disability is shrouded in stigmatization and lack of awareness. Moreover, such a communication can be perceived as an insult to some parents, and they might want to blame someone. It is challenging for parents to accept that their child would now be 'labelled' for his lifetime, thereby dampening the dreams of their child along with their own hopes and aspirations.
- **Be open in your discussion.** It is essential to keep the parents involved from the beginning. Developing a rapport

with the parents and displaying honest and mutual concern for the child, helps in connecting with them, so that they become more receptive to your observations and suggestions.

- **Avoid labelling.** Rather than labelling the child yourself, discuss the child's behaviour with the parents/caregivers, focussing on the symptoms which have been observed.
- **Be patient.** Address the concerns of the parents with patience without getting judgemental, and inform them about the help available. Discuss with them the varied options and available courses of action, and what kind of improvement they must expect. You might have to face repetitive questions, but you should remain calm, as it is important to reduce the parents' anxiety and clarify all their doubts adequately.
- **Provide reassurance**. Educate the parents about their child's intellectual disability and its related concerns while clarifying the questions and doubts that need to be addressed.
- **Bust myths.** There are certain myths and misconceptions concerning individuals with intellectual disabilities and it becomes essential to dispel some of them in order to provide these children with the right kind of effective help.

### Busting Myths Related to Intellectual Disability

**People with intellectual disability are not capable of thinking or doing anything constructive**

People with intellectual disability have different levels of functioning. Every individual has the ability to learn something depending upon their level of intellectual functioning.

**Such people are cursed, punished by God or possessed by demons**

Intellectual disability could be a result of various genetic, environmental, prenatal, or postnatal factors. There is no other factor which is responsible for the problem.

> **Intellectual disability and mental illness are the same**
> Intellectual disability is not an illness. It is not something that can be treated or cured, but with appropriate intervention and education, the children can be helped to be independent to varying degrees.
>
> **Children with intellectual disability are incapable of having feelings or emotions**
> Although they may not be able to express them as expected by the society, but they do have feelings like other people; they do have emotional needs for love, happiness and nurturance.

## STEP 3: Encourage help-seeking and provide information

After talking to the child's parents/caregivers, it is also necessary to show them the path forward. You can reassure them by providing the complete and correct information about the various courses of action needed towards intervention.

Children with intellectual disability require adequate medical and psychological intervention, and hence the role of professional help is irreplaceable. Consultations with a psychiatrist as well as a clinical psychologist would be necessary to develop **Individualized Educational Programs** (IEPs), which are usually tailor-made according to each child's specific needs. Most children would benefit from a combination of special education, occupational therapy, speech therapy, as well as family therapy. The goal of such interventions is to identify the child's strengths and weaknesses, and to work towards fulfilling the child's potential for development. Skill-building is a major component of intervention with intellectual disability, including social-skills, self-help as well as life-skills training.

## STEP 4: Encourage parental involvement

Intervention for intellectual disability is not possible without the involvement of parents, as the child needs to be monitored as well as regulated in all settings. This is only possible when the parent/caregiver works in close tandem with the teacher or the community worker or any other professional working with him. Besides the training and remediation provided by experts, the parents/caregivers also need to be trained to be able to manage the child at home. Moreover, it is quite common for children with intellectual disability to exhibit behavioural difficulties. Therefore, besides skills-building, behavioural management is also an important component of intervention. It is important not only for you to be aware of some such interventional strategies, but also to encourage the parents or the caregivers towards their application at home.

- **Shaping.** To teach any skill or behaviour to an intellectually disabled child, the activity should be broken down into smaller and sequential steps, each being isolated from the other, described and demonstrated to the child one by one. Avoid any punitive measures. Corrective feedback should be given, along with step-by-step rewards for accomplishing each sub-unit.
- **Prompting.** Children with intellectual disability are required to be physically guided to perform skills, which are being shaped, as it speeds up the acquisition of new skills and overall learning.
- **Use a reward system.** Especially when dealing with intellectual disability, rewards and reinforcements need to be used wisely in order to be effective in modifying the child's behaviour. An example of an effective reward system is utilizing token economy, which allows children and adolescents to earn privileges, praise, peer recognition or recognition from parents. It is important to ensure that

the reward system is simple and easily understood by the child as well as the parent or caregiver.

## STEP 5: Building resilience

Intervention is a continuous process when it comes to working in the area of intellectual disability. The level, frequency and intensity of the intervention may wax and wane over time. This makes it important to keep working towards building the individual's resilience towards the problems they may encounter.

- **Encourage sensitivity.** Children with intellectual disability are often the target of ridicule and disappointment among their friends and family. It is important for you to encourage sensitivity in other people, to help make the child's reintegration into society as smooth as possible.
- **Promote social-skills training.** Continued efforts should be made to help the child build good relationships with friends and family. It requires teaching the child skills related to specific social situations using the methods of behaviour modification.
- **Rehabilitation.** Such children should be encouraged to engage in vocational training activities which can also be financially viable depending upon the developmental level of the child and the severity of his disability. This in turn will provide a boost to their self-esteem helping them lead lives which are more independent and self-reliant.
- **Liaison with parents/caregivers.** It is essential to maintain contact with the parents and if possible with the mental health professional treating the child to ensure that regular and consistent follow-ups are being done with regard to the child's progress.

Intellectual disability impacts multiple areas of a child's life and his future. The need for early intervention cannot be emphasized enough to ensure the child progressively develops skills for life. Parental involvement and environmental supports remain critical for the child throughout his life.

# 17
# SPECIFIC LEARNING DISABILITY

As individuals who work closely with children and adolescents, you may come across individuals who appear to have the potential to achieve but are yet not able to get the results that would reflect that potential. Frequently, the adults around them might assume that this is happening because the child is not interested or is lazy or just does not pay attention. What is not looked at is the possibility that the child may be having deficits in learning or what are known as a **specific learning disability** which may be interfering with his performance and reflecting as poor academic results.

## Understanding specific learning disability

It is important to know and recognize that specific learning disabilities are neurodevelopmental disorders which create a difficulty in the child's ability to efficiently perceive and process verbal and non-verbal information. It prohibits them from applying the basic skills relating to reading, writing or mathematics to the process of learning which significantly affects their academic achievement. These deficits which are seen are typically inconsistent with the overall intellectual ability that is demonstrated by the child and can be baffling to the adults around him.

The problems which can indicate towards the presence of a specific learning disability can begin to be noticed in early childhood. However, a complete and comprehensive assessment and diagnosis can only be made once formal education has started. Usually, children who suffer from a specific learning disability tend to find it difficult to keep up with their peers. This may not be the case with all subjects. These children can perform well in some subjects and do rather poorly in others.

The children who are diagnosed with a specific learning disability typically show deficits in one or more of the following areas:

- Reading words or sentences
- Comprehension
- Spellings
- Written expression
- Mathematical calculations
- Mathematical reasoning or word problems

It is also essential to remember that these problems need to manifest for at least a six months period before a diagnosis can be made. The challenge with specific learning disability lies not just in the lack of skills but also the impact that it has on the child in terms of his sense of self as well as his relationships with family and at school. This makes it imperative that you have a good working knowledge and understanding of what these are and what you can do to take care of a child who may have the problem.

### Facts

It is important to understand the prevalence of the condition and other statistical facts associated with it as it is easy to underestimate the rates at which the problem exists among young children and adolescents that you work with.

- Current estimates place the prevalence of specific learning disability at 10 per cent of the youth population (Saddock, Saddock & Ruiz, 2015).
- It occurs 2–3 times more commonly in males than in females (Saddock, Saddock & Ruiz, 2015).
- Adolescents with the problem are 1.5 times more likely to drop out of school, approximating rates of 40 per cent (Saddock, Saddock & Ruiz, 2015).

### How can you identify specific learning disability?

There are numerous indicators which can hint towards the presence of a problem of specific learning disability. Your knowledge and vigilance regarding these aspects can go a long way in ensuring that the child receives timely help to be able to overcome the problem. The following signs can help you to identify a child with the problem at the earliest.

| Warning Signs of Specific Learning Disability |
|---|
| • Poor word recognition |
| • Slow reading rate |
| • Difficulty in comprehending instructions |
| • Challenges in speech sound processing skills |
| • Difficulty in word recognition |
| • Problem in using phonetics to sound out words |
| • Continuous mistakes in spellings |
| • Difficulty in sequencing words |
| • Difficulty in remembering number names and signs |
| • Problem translating word problems into computation |
| • Significant grammatical errors |
| • Not being able to organize a paragraph properly |
| • Poor handwriting |

## What causes a specific learning disability?

The factors that have been implicated in the causation and development of specific learning disabilities include the following.

*Genetic factors:*

Specific learning disorder (SLD) is neurobiological disorder with a strong genetic contribution. There is evidence to suggest that children who have SLD with impairment in reading and written expression have first degree relatives with similar difficulties.

*Neurobiological factors:*

Neurological deficits in areas of the brain responsible for processing sounds of speech, comprehension, spelling, and visual-spatial information may be implicated in SLD. Research in neuroscience and neuropsychology indicates that encoding processes and working memory are problem areas for children with SLD.

*Birth and delivery related factors:*

Complications during pregnancy are common in the histories of children with SLD. Extremely low birth weight and severely premature children are also at an increased risk. Prenatal exposure to maternal infectious illness, such as influenza and perinatal injuries may contribute to SLD. Children malnourished for long periods during early childhood are at an increased risk of poor cognitive performance. Conditions such as lead poisoning, foetal alcohol syndrome, and in utero drug exposure can also be causative factors.

## Why is early intervention required?

It is important to recognize that a specific learning disability responds very well to treatment or intervention. The earlier the problem is identified the sooner the results can be seen in terms of skill acquisition and reduction in the gap between a child's abilities and intellectual capacities and their academic performance. For a child who is diagnosed with a specific learning disability it is possible he needs specialized instructions by a **Special Educator** or the utilization of alternate methods of being taught the same concepts. However, none of these will happen till you as the adult who is closely associated and working with children is able to pick on the signs of the problem at the earliest.

Finally, specific learning disabilities significantly impact a child's levels of motivation and their drive to achieve. If the child is not aware of his problem and does not realize that there are effective solutions he will start viewing his future as bleak. This can impact their interpersonal relationships and interactions with peers. This takes away from a child's thoughts about his own self as being adequate and capable to negotiate the world, impacting his self-esteem, levels of confidence and even self-worth.

**These multiple aspects in their totality make it imperative that early identification and intervention be encouraged and solicited in the case of specific learning disabilities.**

## Who is at risk?

Like any other problem relating to mental health there are certain factors which tend to increase the chances of a child developing a specific learning disability. Given the need for early intervention in this condition, a good working knowledge of these risk factors can help ensure your vigilance in determining the presence of the problem at the earliest.

| Red Flags (Beware As These Increase Risk) |
|---|
| • Significant maternal illness or injury.<br>• Drug or alcohol use during pregnancy.<br>• Maternal malnutrition.<br>• Premature or prolonged labour.<br>• Low birth weight and oxygen deprivation.<br>• Traumatic injuries in childhood.<br>• Severe nutritional deprivation.<br>• Exposure to poisonous substances. |

**The FSMH steps**

**STEP 1: Identify the child at risk**

The first and foremost step is identifying the child who may be at risk for being affected by the condition. Like we have discussed earlier in the chapter, there are numerous early signs that can be observed by you as the adult which could help you identify the presence of the problem at the earliest. Besides the signs which have been discussed previously, the following are additional aspects which should be kept in mind when you are suspecting a specific learning disability with impairment in reading, writing, or mathematics.

**Characteristics of children with SLD with impairment in reading:**

- Deficit in processing sound of speech sound.
- Challenge in identifying parts of words that denote specific sounds.
- Difficulty in recognizing words.
- Difficulty in sounding out words.
- Errors of omission or addition.

- Distortion of words.
- Difficulty in distinguishing between printed letter characters and sizes.
- Slow reading speed.
- Difficulty in sequencing words properly.
- Dislike and avoidance of reading.

## Characteristics of children with SLD with impairment in written expression:

- Problem in spelling out words.
- Difficulty in expressing thoughts.
- Large number of grammatical errors.
- Challenges in organizing paragraphs.
- Comfort in writing in short sentences.
- Failure to capitalize the first letter of the sentence.
- Forgetting to end the sentence with a period.
- Poor handwriting.
- Erroneous word choices.
- Refusal to do written-work at school or home.

## Characteristics of children with SLD with impairment in mathematics:

- Difficulty learning numbers.
- Difficulty in remembering signs for addition, multiplication, etc.
- Challenge in learning multiplication tables.
- Problem in translating word problems to computations.
- Slow pace of performing calculations.
- Challenge in understanding concepts such as counting or adding.
- Difficulty in envisioning clusters of objects as groups.
- Trouble associating auditory and visual symbols.

- Problem in choosing principles for problem-solving activities.

## STEP 2: Rule out any other coexisting condition

Specific learning disabilities have been found to be associated with other coexisting conditions which can make it difficult to treat the condition. It is essential that you develop a good understanding of whether there are any other coexisting conditions such as ADHD, oppositional defiance, conduct disorder, anxiety, or depression. The presence of any of these conditions would complicate the treatment process as all problems need to be taken care of. It would, thus, be advisable to seek comprehensive information from various sources including the child's community, family and school before you begin any conversations with the child or his parents/caregivers.

## STEP 3: Begin a non-confrontational conversation

It is important to remember that most children who have been experiencing significant academic difficulties on account of a specific learning disability which has not been identified yet, would have been subjected to ridicule and criticism by multiple adults and peers in their life. As you approach a child who you suspect has the disability, it is essential that you keep the following aspects in mind for your first conversation with him:

- **Be empathetic in your approach.** The child you are approaching would need to feel that you can understand the difficulty the situation presents for him. It would be important to be able to show him that you are making an effort to be able to see things from his perspective and that you are not coming in with your presumptions into the situation.
- **Listen to the child.** As adults, we frequently want to discuss what we think is happening. In the process, we can forget

to listen to what the child has to say. He may have his own thoughts and feelings about what is happening and before you share what you believe is happening you need to hear him first.
- **Do not attempt to confront him.** The child would not be in a position to enter into a confrontation regarding the views he holds. If he seems to be defensive then do not attempt to tell him what you think is happening. Instead you should communicate your concern and your honest desire to try and help him through the challenges he is facing.
- **Provide him reassurance.** Even if the child does not want to know what exactly it is that may be happening with him, he would still benefit from hearing that things can get better. It is important that you communicate the same to him and help allay his anxieties regarding his future.

## STEP 4: Provide information to the parents/caregivers

It is essential that the parents/caregivers of the child be provided with the right information regarding the problem their child is having which is affecting his academic performance and achievements at school. Regardless of whether this is a problem which is solvable, the parents of a child could potentially have a negative reaction to the diagnosis. The following are somethings you must keep in mind while communicating with the child's parents regarding specific learning disability.
- **Be careful not to use the label.** Instead talk in terms of the deficits that you have observed in child's reading, writing, or maths abilities which you believe may be causing the child to not learn at an adequate level as per his age and grade.
- **Enlist the child's strengths** besides discussing and sharing the deficits you have been noticing. This would help ensure that the parents understand you have a balanced view of

how the child is doing.
- **Use simple language** to communicate and share with the parents about what specific learning disabilities are.
- **Help the parents understand that there is a way to work with a child** who has been diagnosed with the disability and that the problem can be tackled with intervention at the earliest.
- **Bust the myths** that the parents may have in relation to what learning disabilities are, how they are caused and the impact they can have on a child's future.

| Busting Myths Related to Specific Learning Disabilities |
|---|
| **SLD is the same as intellectual deficiency** |
| Learning disorder impedes the ability of the child to learn or use specific academic skills (e.g. reading, writing, or arithmetic), that are required for other academic learning. The learning difficulties are 'unexpected' since other aspects of development and functioning seem to be fine. However, a diagnosis of learning disorder is not always indicative of low intelligence. In fact, some children with learning difficulties display superior creativity. |
| **Excessive use of gadgets causes learning disorder** |
| Learning disorder is a neurodevelopmental condition that cannot be caused by use of gadgets, social networking, or even bad parenting. |
| **People with learning disorder cannot learn** |
| Individuals with a diagnosis of learning disorder have different ways of learning information. Typically, they do not respond well to the traditional classroom instruction method of teaching and learning. |
| **Learning disorder is an excuse for being lazy** |
| Children having learning disabilities often have to work harder than others and yet their results often do not reflect their efforts. It is for this reason that they may become discouraged from time to time, thereby seeming unmotivated or lazy. |

> **Everyone outgrows their learning disorder by adulthood**
> Learning disorder is most likely to be noticed in school; however, the effects range in all areas of life. Usually by adulthood, people find ways to use their strengths to compensate for their learning disabilities. As an example, many adults seek work environments that are a good fit.

## STEP 5: Direct the parent/caregiver to the right expert

When communicating with the parents the essential next step would be to direct them to the right expert who would be able to help them more comprehensively understand the problem and also work towards resolving it. The first expert you would need to refer to would be a clinical psychologist to assess for the presence of the problem using a comprehensive battery of tests. Post the determination of the diagnosis and the confirmation of the presence of a specific learning disability you would need to help the parents locate and work with a **Special Educator** to help the child enhance and develop the skills that are deficient and also to ensure that he is able to start achieving as per his potential. The special educator would work through a specialized **Individualized Education Plan** that would be devised as per the needs of the child and he or she would also involve the parents in helping ensure that some tasks and strategies are undertaken at home as well to ensure the generalization of the skills that are being learnt.

## STEP 6: Inform the parents that the child can receive exemptions and assistance from the education board.

It would be important to inform the parents that their child can receive exemptions for certain subjects and certain assistance such as increased time for giving an examination, provision of an amanuensis, help in understanding a question paper, to name a few—in case the child has a diagnosis of specific learning disability. These exemptions can be availed against the report provided by a clinical psychologist who holds an MPhil degree in clinical psychology and is registered with the Rehabilitation Council of India. This knowledge is essential as it would also enable the parents to recognize that there are ways and methods through which the child's academic life can be made better and which would allow the child to achieve his potential.

### STEP 7: Build resilience post the intervention

The intervention in the case of a specific learning disability can continue for a long time, even lasting for years as the child may require continued support in developing methods of doing his academic tasks. In such a scenario your role becomes even more important as the child would require your continued support in negotiating his environment, both at school with peers and in the community in which he resides. Following are some aspects that you must keep in mind in working with a child who is or has undergone a longitudinal intervention for specific learning disability:

- **Reinforce that the child is no less than anyone** else on account of his learning disability or because he is required to be exempt from some subjects or take the benefits of the relaxations provided by the board of education.
- **Share and discuss in the school and the community** about what learning disabilities are to ensure that there are no misconceptions regarding the problem.
- **Highlight that success in life is also contingent upon hard work and effort** and that the child should focus upon these aspects and not feel let down by the deficits he has today.

- **Encourage the child to work towards his strengths** and also focus on tasks other than those that are academic. Focussing on extracurricular activities would also allow for the development of the child's confidence and belief in his self.
- **Help the child determine other avenues of success** by giving him responsibilities in the classroom.
- **Encourage the child to share and discuss his thoughts, feelings and experiences.** Frequently, children with a specific learning disability can be hesitant in discussing what they go through and this can cause a lot of other problems to emerge such as low moods or anger and irritability as well.
- **Focus on the child's achievements** and highlight the same to help him recognize the changes that are happening and the progress he is making.
- **Help the child build skills relating to social interactions** and provide for greater opportunities to engage in social situations.
- **Help the child to be more assertive** and to stand up for himself as these children can often be victims of bullying at school or within the community.
- **Help the child develop important life skills such as those relating to planning, problem-solving, decision-making and negotiating,** which are critical to success later in life.
- **Help the child focus on what he would want to do ahead in life** so that he can also look towards the steps he needs to plan and take in order to reach his goal.

Difficulty in academic performance can become a significant source of distress for most children. Recognition that this can be on account of a mental health illness can help delineate a precise path for the child to help cope with the problem and build the right skills.

# 18

# AUTISM SPECTRUM DISORDER

Over the years that you have been working with children and adolescents you may have come across children who tend to have very idiosyncratic ways of doing things and eccentricities in their behaviour. You may describe these children as being odd in their behaviour and this may be reflected in the way in which their social relationships and communication patterns are structured as well as in the presence of repetitive behaviour. These groups or categories of behaviour are typically placed under the umbrella term of **Autism Spectrum Disorder**. Understanding the presence of such behaviour and knowing that these may represent problems in development is very critical in how one deals with them.

## Understanding autism spectrum disorder

Autism spectrum disorder (ASD) is a neurodevelopmental disorder which is seen in a spectrum or along a continuum where the core problems are seen to reside in deficits in social communication and in the presence of restricted and repetitive behaviour to varying degrees. This condition typically can be seen by the second year of life and in cases where the symptoms are rather severe, a lack of developmentally appropriate interest in social interactions can be seen as early as the first year of life.

In cases where the symptoms are much milder the diagnosis may not be made for several years.

Children who receive a diagnosis of autism spectrum disorder tend to have a very narrow range of interest in activities. They do not like change and resist it rather strongly. Their responses to the social environment are not in accordance with what is typically seen in their peers of a similar age who do not have the diagnosis. They can display oddities in behaviour and repetitive actions in the form of flapping of hands, toe walking or odd play.

## Facts

- Current prevalence rates estimate the disorder to be present in 1 per cent of the population of children (Saddock, Saddock & Ruiz, 2015).
- The onset of the disorder is in the early developmental period and can be seen as early as 18 months of age.
- Autism spectrum disorder is diagnosed 4 times more often in boys than in girls (Saddock, Saddock & Ruiz, 2015).
- Girls with autism spectrum disorder more often display intellectual disability than boys (Saddock, Saddock & Ruiz, 2015).

## How can you identify autism spectrum disorder?

Identifying autism spectrum disorder at the earliest is rather important. There are some signs the presence of which can communicate the existence of the disorder. It is imperative that you be aware of these warning signs, as early identification is crucial to the success of the intervention in the case of this disorder.

| **Warning Signs of Autism Spectrum Disorder** |
|---|
| • Delayed language development. |
| • Repetition of words or sentences. |
| • Repetitive movements like hand flapping, waving, walking on toes, etc. |
| • Preoccupation with certain objects. |
| • Difficulty in changing routines. |
| • Over-sensitivity to pain, loud noise, or sharp light and touch. |
| • Difficulty in expressing emotions. Not liking hugging others. |
| • Not making eye contact. |
| • Impairment in intellectual functioning. |
| • Lack of pretend play or make-believe play. |

## What causes autism spectrum disorder?

There are multiple factors, the presence of which has been implicated in the development of autism spectrum disorder. The following points take a close look at some of these factors.

*Genetic factors:*

Family and twin studies suggest a significant heritable contribution in autism spectrum disorder. Increased rates of autism, as high as 50 per cent, are seen in siblings of a child with the illness. The siblings are also at a high risk of developing various developmental impairments. The concordance rate is higher in monozygotic twins than in dizygotic twins.

*Immunological factors:*

The lymphocytes of some autistic children have been found to react with maternal antibodies that increases the chances of neural damage of the foetus during gestation which can cause the development of autism spectrum disorder.

*Birth and delivery related factors:*

The most significant prenatal factors associated with ASD are advanced maternal and paternal age at birth, maternal gestational bleeding, gestational diabetes and first born baby. Perinatal risk factors include umbilical cord complications, birth trauma, foetal distress, low birth weight, small for gestational age, congenital malformation, ABO blood group system, or Rh factor incompatibility. Obstetrical complications that are associated with risk of ASD include hypoxia.

## Why is early intervention important?

For any mental health problem which has a developmental aspect associated with it, the need for early intervention cannot be stressed enough. The autism spectrum disorders are one such category of mental health problems seen in children which pertains to development and the earlier an intervention is engaged in the better the results. Chances of a child acquiring some functions or being able to cope with his challenging behaviour are better if the intervention starts at the earliest possible age. This would also ensure that rapid work can be done utilizing the child's strengths. At the same time, early intervention would ensure that you and any other adults working with the child are able to understand things fully and also know what to do and how to do things. It is important to know and remember that the problems that are seen in children with ASD can be identified as early as 18 months of age. Making sure that the child is receiving the right support and intervention which is specific to his challenges on account of autism is a must. The later an intervention starts in the case of ASD the more difficult it is to help the child bring about necessary changes and adaptations. **Thus, the importance and value of an early intervention in the case of autism spectrum disorders can be stressed enough.**

## Who is at risk?

Autism spectrum disorders are challenging to deal and work with. It is important to know that the presence of certain conditions can increase the chances of a child being born with ASD. Your knowledge and understanding of these risk factors is critical in ensuring that the parent/caregiver can be made aware of the need for being more vigilant and aware of their child's development such that in case some symptoms do appear the intervention can be done at the earliest.

### Red Flags (Beware As These Increase Risk)
- Genetic disorders such as Fragile X syndrome and Tuberous Sclerosis.
- Children with a sibling who has ASD.
- Usage of certain prescription medications during pregnancy.
- Children born to older parents.
- Exposure to heavy metals and other toxins in the environment.

## The FSMH steps

### STEP 1: Identify the child at risk

The most important first step in the case of autism spectrum disorders is the identification of the child who is at risk and has the disorder. It is essential for you to be able to identify the problem at the earliest and for doing so it is important for you to be aware of some more signs which could indicate towards the presence of the condition, besides those listed previously in the chapter. These include the following:

- Poor eye contact.
- Repetitive behaviour or movements.
- Preoccupation with specific objects.

- Interest in a limited number of things.
- Inappropriate social interactions.
- Excessive sensitivity to stimuli like lights or sounds.
- Lack of empathy.
- Difficulty in understanding the emotions of the other.

## STEP 2: Share your concerns with the parent/caregiver

If you have been able to determine that a child may be showing the symptoms of autism spectrum disorders, the next step would be to share your knowledge with the parents/caregivers of the child. You as the adult who is working with the child would need to engage and involve the parents in this process if an intervention is to be done. Following are some aspects that must be kept in mind when sharing your understanding of the possibility of the presence of ASD in a child:

- **Be mindful of the language you use** in sharing your concerns with the parent, it would be imperative that you do not use jargon and complicated language to share what you are suggesting is happening.
- **Talk about the things you have been noticing in terms of the behaviour the child is displaying,** his communication patterns and social interactions. Do not be in a hurry to state that you think the child may be having ASD.
- **Develop an understanding of what the parents' experience has been with the child.** Elicit their concerns and the problems they have been observing or having trouble coping with.
- **Be empathic and show your concern for the child,** particularly his future and ability to achieve up to his potential on account of the difficulties he has been experiencing.
- **Do not sound like you are panicking.** The child's parents may be feeling very lost and unsure of what they need to

do. If you sound like you are panicking or unsure then this would only serve to increase the parent's anxiety.
- **Take control of the situation and lead the conversation.** Do not allow the disclosure of the problems to unravel the situation into a chaotic experience. You need to follow to the next step which is to disclose the suspected diagnosis and direct the parents to the right experts.

## STEP 3: Help the parent make sense of the problem

For a large majority of the parents whose children get diagnosed with the autism spectrum disorders, understanding the illness can be rather difficult. After you have helped the parents understand and accept that there is a problem which needs to be tackled, it is your role to help them develop a more cogent understanding of the problem. The first aspect of this is to help the parents know and understand that this is an illness like any other and it does not relate to anything that they may have or have not done. At the same time it is essential that you help the parent recognize that a lot of the symptoms the child displays are not in his voluntary control and are a part of the illness. As a result, continuously pushing the child to be different or penalizing him for his behaviour will be of no help. It is essential that after you have shared with the parents your knowledge of the disorder you also help dislodge some of the common myths and assumptions that are associated with the problem.

---

**Busting Myths Related to Autism Spectrum Disorders**

**Children with autism have intellectual deficiency**

Often times, autism brings with it just as many exceptional abilities as limitations. Many children with autism have been found to have normal to high IQs. In fact, some children may even excel at math, music, or any other pursuit.

| |
|---|
| **Children with autism can't understand others' emotions** |
| Autism often affects an individual's ability to understand unspoken interpersonal communication. Due to this, children diagnosed with autism spectrum disorder might not be able to detect sadness based solely on one's body language or sarcasm in one's tone of voice. However, a more direct communication of emotions makes it easier for children with autism to feel empathy and compassion for others. |
| **Autism is caused by bad parenting** |
| Originating in the 1950s, a theory known as the 'refrigerator mother hypothesis' arose and gained popularity which suggested that autism was caused by mothers who lacked emotional warmth. This theory has long been disproved. |
| **Children with autism don't feel emotions** |
| Children with autism spectrum disorder are highly capable of feeling emotions and love. However, they have problems with emotional expression and communication. Even though this is one of the most common characteristics of ASD, children can build skills in this area and learn to respond to other people more appropriately. |
| **Children with autism don't want friends and want to be alone** |
| The above said might not always be true. Recent research has found that while some individuals diagnosed with ASD might want to have friends and be social, they do not know the appropriate ways of doing it. Since understanding and appropriately responding to people's emotions might also be an issue, dealing with social situations may make them uncomfortable. |

## STEP 4: Encourage help-seeking from the right experts

It is critical in a problem like ASD that help be sought from the right experts. Besides having a discussion with the child's paediatrician it will be important for the parents to meet with a psychiatrist as well as a psychologist to reach the right diagnosis as well as for a comprehensive assessment and evaluation of the exact nature of the problem, its intensity, and range of functions that it affects for the child. Based on the results that are generated, typically the child will need to be referred to other experts such as an applied behaviour analyst, an occupational therapist or an art-based therapist. The decision of which expert would eventually work with the child would be contingent upon the results of the analysis.

## STEP 5: Prepare the parents for the longitudinal course of the illness

In most cases where there is a diagnosis of ASD the intervention is a continuous process as at each stage and phase of life new challenges can emerge and new skills may need to be focused on. It is important that you explain and re-emphasize to the parents that ASD is not a treatable problem. The experts working with the child will be able to mitigate some of the problems, enhance the adaptation to others, while building skills in some areas. However, a complete cure is not possible. This can be a rather distressing and challenging reality for parents to cope with. It would be your role to ensure that the parent is able to work through his grief and sense of distress as well as lack of surety about the future for the child as that would be a crucial aspect for the child's overall adjustment to his life.

## STEP 6: Build resilience post the intervention

There may or may not be an end point to the interventions and it is possible that the course of intervening can wax and wane over time. It is going to be important to take care of some additional aspects relating to the child's self and environment to ensure his overall well-being.

- **Build comprehensive knowledge about the problem the child is experiencing in the minds of all other adults** besides the primary caregivers who may be dealing with the child. This could be his teachers, relatives, or any other significant adults.
- **Focus on the things the child can do** and not on the things he is not being able to accomplish for himself.
- **Do not push the child in a direction that he is not keen to explore.** Children with ASD can have idiosyncratic ways of doing things and they frequently do not like things to be shaken out of their routine.
- **Work with what the child is comfortable with.** Gently encourage him to explore the limits of his boundaries.
- **Help the child engage in activities** whether academic or extracurricular in an area that is of interest to him.
- **Stay continuously connected with both his family and the experts** working with the child.

Autism spectrum disorder requires the continued intervention and support from multiple professionals and the adults who surround the child. Criticism and punitive measures do not help resolve the deficits which are characteristic of the illness. Instead a problem solving approach that seeks to tackle the symptoms that emerge as a part of the constellation of the illness along with focus on specific long-term goals is the best way forward.

# 19

# TRAUMA AND ABUSE

Our lives are filled with various significant experiences, both positive and negative. While we enjoy and savour the positive ones, the negative experiences, too, have significant and long-lasting effects on our lives. These negative experiences range from daily life struggles to more severe and intense negative experiences which can be rather difficult to deal with.

**Trauma** refers to any severe psychological or physiological stressor which results in damaging effects to an individual. It includes events such as experience of rape, abuse, natural disasters resulting in loss of life and property, to name a few. Such experiences differ in quality from other negative experiences in their capacity to overwhelm one's ability to cope with what has happened. Abuse (physical, sexual, or emotional) is one such significant experience which can result in childhood trauma. **Child abuse** refers to any form of physical, mental and sexual exploitation of or cruelty towards a child by a parent or other adult, causing significant harm to the child. **Neglect** of a child's needs by a parent also constitutes abuse and can have a similar impact.

Traumatic experiences can be short-lived, that is, occurring at a single period of time, such as natural disasters, serious accidents, or may occur repeatedly over a long period of time, such as continuous physical or sexual abuse, or neglect.

## Facts

- 25-90 per cent children, who have been exposed to some form of trauma (environmental events, abuse, or neglect) develop significant mental health issues (Saddock, Saddock & Ruiz, 2015).
- Children who have been exposed to trauma repeatedly or for a long duration are at greater risk for developing mental health issues (Saddock, Saddock & Ruiz, 2015).
- In India, 5 to 12-year-olds have reported higher levels of abuse than other age groups (UNICEF, 2007).
- 2 out of 3 children are physically abused (UNICEF, 2007).
- 53 per cent children have experienced sexual abuse of one form or another (UNICEF, 2007).
- Boys and girls are at an equal risk of abuse (UNICEF, 2007).
- Persons in trust or positions of authority are major abusers (UNICEF, 2007).
- 70 per cent of children, who experience abuse and resulting trauma, never report the matter to anyone (UNICEF, 2007).

As these events are mostly under-reported, adequate and timely help is not always able to reach those who need it, particularly in the underprivileged segments of the society. These statistics depict the urgency and need for focussing attention on child abuse and trauma and providing timely and appropriate intervention.

## What are the different forms that abuse can take?

### Physical abuse

Physical abuse refers to all those activities which are done deliberately with an intention to physically hurt or injure a child, such as beating, slapping, pinching, to name a few. These acts, not only physically hurt the child, but also have an impact on their psychological well-being and their overall sense of safety.

*Sexual abuse*

Child sexual abuse refers to the use of a child for sexual gratification, by an adult. It involves forcing or enticing a child or young person to take part in sexual activities, including prostitution, whether or not the child is aware of what is happening. The activities may involve physical contact (penetrative or non-penetrative acts) and also include non-contact activities, such as involving children in looking at, or in the production of, pornographic material or watching sexual activities, or encouraging children to behave in sexually inappropriate ways.

*Emotional abuse and neglect*

Emotional abuse and neglect refer to child maltreatment through certain parenting practices which results in adverse consequences for the child. While emotional abuse is intentional in nature, neglect is non-intentional. Emotional abuse involves activities such as frequent punishment even for minor faults, frequent rejection or humiliation, to name a few.

## Signs and symptoms of trauma and abuse

Child abuse and trauma can manifest in both externalizing and internalizing symptoms. That is a child may act out, become violent, aggressive, abuse other children, or the child may become withdrawn, depressed and become increasingly fearful and anxious. Some signs that show the child is a victim of abuse and resultant trauma include:

- Loss of interest in activities.
- Regular physical complaints such as headaches or stomach aches.

- Extreme emotional reactions.
- Trouble sleeping.
- Irritability, anger, or violence.
- Difficulty in concentrating.
- Constant or often clingy behaviour
- Regression to a younger age.
- Increased vigilance or alertness to the environment.
- Refusal to go to or to be around specific places or people.

In addition to these symptoms, extreme and recurring negative experiences or abuse can result in the child developing **Post-traumatic Stress Disorder (PTSD)**, exhibiting symptoms, in addition to those mentioned above, such as:

1. Re-experiencing of the traumatic event through intrusive, recurring thoughts, or nightmares.
2. Avoiding situations or people who are associated with the traumatic experience.

These cause significant impairment in the child's life, affecting functioning in home, school and other areas as well. Persistence of these symptoms for more than a month would need professional intervention.

### How can you identify trauma and abuse?

As front-line professional dealing with children, it is important to understand that in most cases abuse and trauma is not reported directly by the victims. The symptoms of trauma and abuse are a manifestation of underlying emotional issues within children, including extreme anxiety and fear, self-blame, feelings of inferiority or shame, feeling threatened by the environment, and it is in the attempt to deal with these negative feelings that child shows certain behaviour, which may point to the presence of trauma and abuse history.

At times, it can be challenging to determine whether a child has been a victim of abuse, as children themselves and family members (especially if the perpetrator is within the family) go to great extents to hide the abuse. Astute observation skills, as well as complete and correct information are, therefore, the most necessary tools for you as the one in direct contact with the child to ensure the timely identification of the problem.

| Warning Signs of Abuse |
| --- |
| • Repeated injury marks. |
| • Easily startled. |
| • Reduced appetite. |
| • Withdrawn behaviour. |
| • Disturbed sleep or nightmares. |
| • Avoiding certain people, family members, or other relatives. |
| • Withdrawal or mistrust of adults. |
| • Excessive secretiveness or irritability. |
| • Complaining about home or family. |
| • Age inappropriate sexual knowledge or behaviour. |
| • Suicidal talk or attempts. |
| • Sudden or drastic change in behaviour. |
| • Avoiding school or home. |
| • Avoiding going to the doctor or for a physical check-up. |
| • Defensive behaviour of child and/or parents when possibility of abuse is discussed. |

The stigma, guilt and shame associated with abuse usually lead children to keep it a secret and not report it, which can make it difficult for a person trying to intervene in the situation. However, it is important to treat a child or teenager affected by the problem with sensitivity while making a special effort to connect with them every day, as victims of abuse experience overwhelming emotions which can have a long-lasting impact.

Also, it is important that necessary steps should be taken to ensure the child's safety by involving the right adults associated with the child or teenager's life. It is very important that the cycle is broken and timely intervention is provided to ameliorate the impact of the event/s.

## What causes or maintains trauma and abuse

While traumatic events, which occur at a single period of time, are beyond an individual's control, the repeated instances of abuse and trauma have certain causal factors which explain their occurrence. There are certain traits which can contribute to the occurrence of abuse and resultant trauma. These can be understood in terms of child-related factors and environmental factors which includes both, the traits of the perpetrator and other factors.

*Child-related factors:*

While there are no specific child factors which cause abuse, there are certain factors which make the child more vulnerable to experience the resultant trauma. These factors include low self-esteem, high sense of guilt, feelings of helplessness, low help-seeking behaviour, proneness to secrecy, poor assertiveness skills, low physical strength, fear of punishment, low self-efficacy and poor coping skills. Although these factors don't contribute to causing abuse; however, they do result in the maintenance of the abusive relationship.

*Environmental or contextual factors:*

These include traits relating to the perpetrator such as a history of being abused themselves, poor self-esteem, cognitive distortions regarding sense of self and view of others, and substance abuse. When the abuser is the parent, marital conflict and discord, dissatisfaction from marriage, poor family support, also contribute to abuse.

## Why is early intervention important?

Considering the fact that victims of abuse, are at higher risk of developing other mental health problems or also becoming abusers themselves, it is very important to break this cycle of abuse. Additionally, abuse requires proper and timely reporting of the incident as it causes significant harm to the child's safety. Children who have been abused are at a higher risk for other comorbid conditions such as mood disorders, anxiety and substance abuse. They are also more likely to indulge in self-harm, have suicidal thoughts and attempts. For these reasons, **it is imperative to be empowered to prevent such adverse outcomes through ensuring identification at the earliest and provision of adequate and timely psychiatric and psychological intervention.**

## Who is at risk?

Regardless of age, gender, caste, religion, or culture, any child can be a victim of abuse and resultant trauma. As a large number of abusive incidents occur at home or within the family, it is very important that front-line professionals and concerned adults outside the family be observant and aware of such possibility and certain behaviour which may serve as red flags.

| Red Flags (Beware As These Increase Risk) |
|---|
| • Marital discord or conflict in parents.<br>• Parent with a history of being abused.<br>• Difficult and challenging family circumstances.<br>• Poor problem-solving skills.<br>• Excessive sense of guilt.<br>• Low sense of self.<br>• Low peer group support and other support mechanisms. |

## The FSMH steps

### STEP 1: Identify the children at risk

Some behavioural signs that you need to watch out for include the following:
- Being suspicious and avoidant of adults.
- Getting irritable and even angry.
- Being defensive.
- Sleep and appetite disturbances.
- Being easily startled.
- Being withdrawn.
- Age inappropriate sexual knowledge or behaviour.
- Lack of attention and concentration.
- Drop in grades and class performance.
- Talking of suicide and suicide attempts.

### STEP 2: Begin a non-confrontational conversation

- **Don't hesitate to begin the conversation.** As someone who has identified a child at risk of being abused and experiencing trauma, you could feel hesitant about broaching the subject, fearing a denial due to the child or adolescent's need to hide the situation. They are often scared to ask for help, and continue struggling internally within themselves. It is of great value to help such children by talking to them, helping them realize that someone does understand and care about what they are feeling and experiencing, and someone is there who they can feel safe with.
- **Be non-confrontational.** It is important to talk to the child in a manner which doesn't make him feel attacked or blamed. Rather, a feeling of support and understanding needs to be communicated by being empathic towards the child's experiences. Always remember that the child's sense

of safety and security has already been compromised, thus, it is of prime importance that he feels safe in talking about the incident with you.
- **Express your concerns about the child's safety.** In cases, where the abuser is someone close to the child, he will not want to report the incident due to attachment to that person or also because of feeling threatened or even guilty. Discuss with the child, the prime importance of their safety, and how it is important that these incidents stop. Help them deal with and reduce their sense of shame and guilt by reducing the tendency towards self-blame.
- **Be reassuring.** Most children and adolescents would be anxious and unsure of the consequences of their speaking out and reaching for help. They need someone to be able to listen to them, empathize and provide reassurance. Do not scare them with the potential consequences of the incident in the long-term. Instead, focus on the possibility of seeking help.

## STEP 3: Encourage help-seeking by involving responsible adults and provide information

As the one who has identified the abuse and trauma being borne by a child or adolescent, it is necessary to involve the parents or the caregivers by informing them about the incident, after explaining to the child the importance and need for the same. It would be common to be faced with parents or caregivers who would be unaware of the abuse that the child has experienced. They may respond with denial and be ashamed or embarrassed about not knowing and may also feel guilty about not having helped the child. It is imperative to handle their anxieties, and help them come to terms with the situation. In your approach with families, keep in mind the following:

- Do not be critical.

- Help them overcome their sense of guilt.
- Help them remove the element of self-blame and anger.
- Encourage them to share their concerns with you.
- Push them to be available for the child without being harsh or intrusive, and giving the child the space to open up at his own pace.
- Enable them to make more sense of the prevailing situation and make them steer away from the how and why for the time being.
- Ensure they understand the consequences of not seeking help from an expert.
- Encourage to seek help for their own selves from family, friends or even a professional, in case they are unable to cope with the knowledge of the circumstances.

As victims of abuse and their caregivers often hesitate in seeking help, it is imperative that they are explained the need for the same. Beyond ensuring the continued safety of the child, the abuse incident requires psychological intervention, frequently warranting the need for psychiatric medications as well. The child needs to be assessed for physical harm and provided appropriate treatment. Explaining to the child and the family the need and importance of seeking help which will also help improve the outcome in the long run. You would need to make them aware of the available healthcare services and other resources, and also encourage and support them for seeking help from the same.

## STEP 4: Reduce stigma and shame

Children who are victims of abuse, particularly sexual abuse, are often guilt-ridden and ashamed about it, which reduces the chance of them seeking help. The stigma associated with having a problem in itself can also be a strong contributing factor to the continued presence of the emotions associated with the traumatic experience. For children who may have experienced a traumatic incident, it is also possible that comparisons made with others and how they are coping with the same or similar situation can make them avoid discussing things even if they are feeling disturbed. It is important to remember that secrecy and hiding only leads to further negative impact to the child's physical and mental health. By reducing the shame and guilt associated, through discussions about the same, you will help the child feel confident about seeking help and ending the abuse or the trauma in his mind.

## STEP 5: Build knowledge to promote prevention

An integral part of working with children and adolescents is the idiom of prevention. To protect them it is important to make them aware of:

- Ways of protecting themselves.
- Identifying that they are experiencing an emotional upheaval or turmoil for which they need help.
- Knowing who they can approach in case they feel they need help.
- At the same time it is important to integrate the following aspects in your interactions as a teacher, counsellor, or parent with children and adolescents:
- Maintaining boundaries.
- Good touch and bad touch.
- Sharing of experiences.
- Dispelling myths that it is a weakness to seek help.
- Reassurance of your consistent presence as a support system.

## STEP 6: Build resilience post the intervention

What happens after intervening in the case of abuse or trauma is as important in helping the child live a better life. Abuse or trauma will continue to remain a significant event in the child's life but it should not be made as the only significant aspect of his life. Seeing and treating the child only as a victim will not help the child in any way. Rather the focus should be on overall functioning and improvement, and building resilience through the following ways:

- **Maintain your interactions with the child the way they were prior** to the episode of abuse or trauma.
- **Educate others around the child about such experiences,** helping them understand that such situations can arise with anyone and, thus, reduce the associated stigma.
- **Express hope and optimism to motivate the child** towards resuming a healthy lifestyle, and encourage his efforts towards the same. Help the child realize that his life will not be defined by one incident alone.
- **Help the child explore his talents to boost his self-confidence** and to shift his focus to more achievement-oriented tasks.
- **Work on the child's sense of self** as such experiences frequently make children doubt their own roles in the causation of the traumatic experience.
- **Help the child break the cycle of guilt and self-blame.** Children frequently in such situations blame themselves for what has happened. It is essential that you keep reiterating that the child had no role to play in the occurrence of the event and it was in no way related to who he is as an individual.
- **Work on helping the child build good relationships** with friends and family as these would form the support systems for the rest of his life.
- **Help the child explore his strengths and the aspects he considers good in his own self.**
- **Assist the child in overcoming difficult emotional experiences and help him see that these are a natural part of life,** while focussing on bridging any deficits in

coping that may be present.
- **Help the child develop mechanisms of reaching out for the future.** This is extremely important so that the child knows what needs to or can be done if there is a similar situation in the future. This would help take away the feeling of helplessness that the child can experience.
- **Maintain contact with the parents and the mental health professional** to ensure that regular and consistent follow-ups are being done.

Trauma and abuse have the capacity to significantly offset the lifecycle of a child and can be very difficult for him to share and discuss. Sensitivity is a crucial first step in reaching out and helping the child stabilize and thereafter a proactive approach to help the child cope and build his supportive structures needs emphasis.

# 20

# SUICIDE AND SELF-HARM

Just the word **suicide** is enough to evoke many powerful images, emotions and even judgements in us. There is tremendous stigma, a sense of fear, apprehension, and a strong silence that is associated with suicide, due to which we frequently hesitate to ask questions or talk about it openly. For a front-line professional, having the correct information about suicide and self-harm, and being aware of the guidelines for prevention, identification and intervention is a must to being empowered to handle children/teens who might be at risk and in need of help.

## Understanding suicide and self-harm

There are many physical and emotional changes that occur during the adolescent years, which along with the challenges that present themselves through the period of growing up, can induce vulnerability, particularly where there are deficits in coping, problem-solving and support mechanisms. When teenagers go through difficult emotions such as loneliness or extremely stressful situations that have grave ramifications on their self-esteem and self-concepts, they can be driven to self-harm or even suicide, especially when there are no protective factors which act as buffers.

A suicidal child is filled with many despairing and negative thoughts and emotions that make it difficult for him to see beyond a very narrowly focussed area. Such children feel helpless about being able to change the present and, therefore, are hopeless about the future and are driven to self-destruction. In fact, helplessness and hopelessness are defining characteristics of the way a suicidal person thinks.

Some teenagers also harbour certain myths about suicide that are sometimes propagated in the media and frequently talked about in their peer group. They might think suicide is an act of bravery or rebellion. At the same time, their sense of identification with their peers can cause them to imitate the act of another—what has been called as **Copycat Suicides or Werther's Syndrome**.

### Facts

- Suicide is the third leading cause of death among teenagers worldwide and this trend continues to rise even today (WHO, 2002).
- About 20 per cent of high school students tend to experience suicidal ideation.
- In the last several decades the number of teen suicides has quadrupled.
- 90 per cent of those who commit suicide have a diagnosable psychiatric condition which if treated on time would have prevented the attempt.
- 70 per cent of those with a diagnosable psychiatric condition who attempt suicide have a mood disorder.

### How can you identify the warning signs of suicide?

It is a myth that suicide is usually an impulsive decision or that it happens on the spur of the moment. Suicide is mostly a well-thought-out decision and there are many clear warning signs that people contemplating suicide typically demonstrate. It is important to be vigilant to these signs, and to know how to respond to them. Not only are there clues about impending suicidal behaviour but there also exist desperate cries for help. Being aware of this fact and changing your perspective about some such behaviour can make you more open, non-judgemental and involved in trying to help the child or adolescent.

If someone talks about self-harm or suicide, it is important to take them seriously and to evaluate the risk factors for the same. Most children who make the following or similar verbal statements might be seriously contemplating self-harm or suicide, particularly if these statements are made with increasing frequency:

- 'I hate my life.'
- 'I wish I could go somewhere and never come back.'
- 'I wish I could sleep and never have to wake up.'
- 'Nothing matters anymore.'
- 'People would be better off without me.'
- 'Life is not worth living.'
- 'I want to kill myself.'
- 'There's no way out.'
- 'It would be better if I were dead.'

There is also certain behaviour that can communicate suicidal intent. It is important that you be on the lookout for such behaviour and treat it seriously.

| Warning Signs of Suicidal Intent |
|---|
| • Indulging in risk-taking behaviour such as reckless driving. |
| • Giving away precious possessions. |
| • Isolating self from family and friends. |
| • Increased alcohol or substance use. |

- Increasing fascination with death/suicide related music, movies and literature.
- Expressing feelings of hopelessness and helplessness.
- Dramatic changes in mood.
- Extreme feelings of anxiety, anger, or revenge.
- A sense of purposelessness in life.
- Looking for lethal or poisonous objects like guns or pills.
- Suicidal talk or attempts.

## The continuum of self-harm and suicide

An adolescent or child who indulges in self-harm or self-injury may or may not be suicidal. It can sometimes be difficult to distinguish between self-injury and a suicide attempt. Regardless of the intent, non-suicidal self-injury also needs to be taken seriously as accidental death can occur and these persons generally require intervention from a trained mental health expert to help them learn better coping behaviour. It is important to recognize that 40 per cent of those who commit suicide have had past attempts at injury and harm to the self (Saddock, Saddock & Ruiz, 2015).

There are many kinds of behaviour that can come under the rubric of self-harm or self-injury. Some of these which you should be wary of and keep a lookout for when working with children and adolescents include—

- Cutting, scratching, or pinching skin such that leaves marks or leads to bleeding.
- Burning one's skin with things such as cigarette butts, incense sticks, or hot water.
- Self-medicating or overdosing on medications or substances.
- Carving on the skin using blades, scissors, or knives.
- Tearing skin.
- Not letting wounds heal.

## Why do children and adolescents injure themselves?

It is difficult and challenging to understand someone who self-injures. There are many adolescents who regularly injure or harm themselves without necessarily wanting to commit suicide, inflicting wounds on their body and also using them to show off to their peers. Such behaviour may frequently appear to be bizarre and incomprehensible to you, making you confront and question them. In fact, this behaviour can continue unabated for several years, without adults around the child/adolescent even realizing that something like this is happening.

Self-harm is a faulty coping mechanism for some people. Children who may be indulging in such behaviour can find it tough to express the intensity of their negative emotions—anger, pain and distress—through words, and feel that physically harming themselves gives them a kind of emotional release. When spoken to, they would not be in a position to explain the reasons and rationale for their behaviour in a coherent and cogent fashion.

On other occasions, the adolescent might feel that he is not able to communicate his thoughts, feelings and the desperation he experiences to a significant other and might find this to be the only language to get their feelings across.

However, the problem with such kind of coping is that it is temporary and the relief associated with it is short lived. This is why the behaviour of causing injury to the self occurs repeatedly each time a situation occurs that is distressing and brings with it difficult and intense emotions. Also, regardless of the intention, children who self-injure are at a higher risk for accidental death, and are vulnerable to developing suicidal ideation. Such a situation needs to be taken very seriously by all the adults around the child/adolescent.

## What causes suicide?

As with any other mental health illness, suicide also finds its underpinnings in various factors which in combination increase the chances of a suicide attempt and even a completed suicide. These include the following:

### Genetic factors:

For children and adolescents with a family history of suicide, particularly in their immediate family, the risk for suicide tends to be 2–4 times higher (Saddock, Saddock & Ruiz, 2015).

### Biological factors:

There is increasing evidence to suggest that both low levels of serotonin and the substrate 5-hydroxyindoleacetic acid (5-HIAA) are implicated in the causation of both impulsivity and aggressive behaviour. These can be considered to cause suicidal attempts and complete suicides as well.

### Psychosocial factors:

Numerous psychosocial factors have been implicated in the causation of suicidal ideation, attempts at suicide and its completion. Aspects like helplessness, hopelessness, worthlessness, impulsivity, substance use, family related disturbances in the form of abuse and violence tend to have a significant impact. It is widely acknowledged that for those who have extremely stressful lives or familial circumstances, resorting to aggression or having suicidal impulses is quite common.

What is most essential to remember is that suicide is not something that happens in a singular moment of impulse or despair unaffected by experiences of the past. There are both proximal and distal factors which are associated with it which create the inclination to engage in some form of self-harm:

*Distal factors:*

By distal factors one would mean those which in the long run tend to create vulnerability in the child or teen to cause some form of self-harm or attempted suicide. These could include factors relating to genetics, family or home environment, personality or individual characteristics, associated long-term stressors, sociocultural variables, to name a few, which could lead to a predisposition on the part of the child/teen to act in a moment of impulse in the future.

*Proximal factors:*

The proximal factors are the triggers or precipitating factors which occur near the attempt of suicide. It could be an experience such as failing an examination or challenges in interpersonal relationships, including the availability of an agent or medium to engage in self-harm which could lead to the actual act of attempting suicide.

## Who is at risk?

It is important to note that suicidal thoughts and feelings can occur in anybody regardless of age, gender, social, or economic and academic background. Children and adolescents can at different points in time entertain thoughts of self-harm and mull over questions relating to death; however, there are certain significant risk factors that make them act on these thoughts and feelings. When a child or adolescent feels so hopeless and sad, that he sees no escape or positive outcome from a stressful situation, he may contemplate suicide.

### Red Flags (Beware As These Increase Risk)

- Family history of suicide.
- Death of a loved one.
- Challenges in interpersonal relationships.
- Dysfunctional family or exposure to family violence.
- Drug or alcohol abuse.
- Depression.
- High levels of hopelessness.
- High levels of impulsivity.
- Previous suicidal attempt.
- Availability of lethal methods.
- Experience of bullying.
- Academic difficulties.
- Isolation from peers.
- Adjustment problems.

## The FSMH steps

### STEP 1: Identify the child at risk

Identify children who may be showing some of the warning signs which may indicate suicidal intent. As discussed above, there are numerous signs and symptoms which make themselves visible before a suicidal attempt is made. It is important to be vigilant and to take these signs seriously. If you do suspect a child to be contemplating suicide it is important that you do not panic. Remember, you have certain steps that you can follow, that are discussed here. Having an action plan helps to deal with the feeling of inadequacy that you may experience in case you have not handled a similar situation before.

If a child comes up to you on his own, be cognizant of the tremendous amount of trust that he has placed in you but also maintain a calm demeanour. This is not the time for you to deal with your own feelings of discomfort or panic, but rather to provide the appropriate help to the child. Regardless of how negative or nihilistic the content of his conversation might be—by coming to you he has shown a clear help-seeking behaviour which is a positive sign and indicates that he doesn't really wish to die.

Also, be vigilant for any conversation that you may overhear which indicates that a child or adolescent is actively engaging in self-harm or is contemplating suicide and do not hesitate to be proactive in reaching out to him.

## STEP 2: Listen and reassure

Most children and adolescents who talk about suicide and send out these warning signs are seeking help and are usually ambivalent about wanting to end their lives. They are blinded by their anger, pain, frustration, or distress, and wish to put a stop to this suffering. But their vision has shrunk to an extent where they see no other way out of their situation. They may have faulty problem-solving and decision-making skills which would be compromising their abilities to cope with the situation. They might also wish for an alternative solution to end their pain, and they simply need to be guided to find a way to continue living. When talking to someone who might be hurting themselves or be suicidal, it is good to remember what that child might be looking for and follow through with **ACT**:

**Absence of judgement:** Such a person is looking for a truly sympathetic ear that does not judge or try to give advice. He would want someone who can understand his problem and does not try to diminish or demean the issue or his distress.

**Care:** Be authentic, sincere and honest. Show that you care and get your concern across to the child clearly. Many suicidal children feel expendable and unwanted. They feel if they were to die no one would miss them. It is of great value to help such children feel like someone cares about what they are feeling and going through.

**Trust:** As a responsible listener you will have to instil trust in the person. This means giving them and their crisis complete respect. At the same time you should never promise a suicidal person complete confidentiality as you will need to inform someone of their intentions in order to help them. However, you may consider involving the person in deciding who (a responsible adult in their lives) can be told.

## STEP 3: Assess for suicide risk

This step will need to be incorporated with Step 2 when you are listening and understanding the child's experience and as a result, gaining his trust and forming a rapport with him.

The two most important questions that ascertain suicide risk are:

- **Does the person have a current plan?**

It is important to ascertain if the child has a plan or has thought deeply enough about the methods he would like to adopt to commit suicide and if he has arranged for the means to do it.

- **Has there been a previous attempt?**

If the child has attempted to commit suicide before, chances are higher that he will be successful in his attempt subsequently.

If you feel that a particular child or teenager is at risk, you can check the risk by direct questioning. It is a myth that talking about suicide increases the risk of suicide. In fact, the taboo surrounding suicide and hesitation to talk about it makes it even harder for the child at risk to share his feelings and intent. Even if you suspect a child to be having suicidal thoughts, it is better to ask because you cannot make a child suicidal by showing that you care. In fact, giving a child a chance to express his feelings can actually provide a release to pent-up negative feelings, and may even prevent a suicide attempt.

You could begin a conversation by indicating that you have been feeling concerned about the child lately and you could also point out the changes you might have observed in the child's behaviour. Once you are able to engage the child in talking about his feelings in an honest and trusting manner, you can ask questions like:

- Do you get thoughts of doing something to yourself or engaging in self-harm?
- How long do you feel you can control acting out on these thoughts?
- Have you made a plan for committing suicide?
- Have you ever tried to engage in any kind of self-harm before?

## STEP 4: Inform the caregiver

If a child is suicidal, it is imperative to inform at least one caregiver. In this case confidentiality is forgone in service to the child's life. Here the priority becomes to keep the child's life out of danger till the crisis passes. The following need to be followed in a regimented way:

- A highly suicidal child should not be left alone.
- The parent also needs to be psycho-educated to detoxify the home. This means that all dangerous items including sharp objects, pills and poisonous substances need to be removed from the reach of the child.
- The child should not be allowed access to the balcony or the terrace either.
- It is absolutely crucial to direct the family to seek help from a psychiatrist at the earliest to prevent any unfortunate incident.

Sometimes, the child at risk might insist that he doesn't mean to kill himself but rather is only indulging in self-harm behaviour for any of the reasons discussed above like emotional release. This may not appear to be a crisis situation; however, such a child requires your help and intervention. This child would be greatly benefitted if he is helped with problem-solving and coping more effectively with situations, thoughts and emotions, which can be done by you or with the help of a mental health professional like a psychologist.

## STEP 5: Guide towards the right help

Suicidal thoughts and intent are very often associated with a treatable mental health illness and such a realization can not only instil a sense of confidence but also make the person in question more amenable to seeking professional help as it generates hope that the problem is solvable. It is important that an adult, with whom the child or teen is comfortable, accompanies him to the required professional, especially for the first session. This could be a psychiatrist, a counsellor, a psychotherapist, or a qualified suicide prevention and crisis intervention centre.

## STEP 6: Instilling resilience post the intervention

Even after the crisis is over, it is important to remember that it is essential to be on your guard and remain involved for a considerable amount of time afterwards.

- **Express hope and optimism** that the child will soon be able to do and perform in the same way that he used to be able to earlier.
- **Give frequent encouragement** and positive strokes.
- **Encourage free expression** and help the child find a safe outlet to vent his thoughts and feelings—whether this is in the form of writing, painting, drama, or role-play.
- **Help the child understand his experience** and identify the

triggers so that he is able to reach out far earlier in case a similar situation presents itself again.
- **Help the child develop an effective support system.** Ensure that the child has sufficient social support both at home and in school.
- **Help the child devise strategies to offset his thoughts** in case he feels suicidal in the future.

## STEP 7: Prevention policy

As an adult working with children, it is important for you to promote active life-skills training in order to help children and adolescents develop healthier coping mechanisms to deal with their internal conflicts. Such policies are a must especially for school children and teenagers. Efforts should be made to focus on building trust and rapport with them, so as to enable an atmosphere of open communication, encouraging the reporting and sharing of their innermost feelings easily. Work on the following aspects which act as protective factors for a child against suicide:

- Provide social-skills training
- Enhance problem-solving
- Work on decision-making
- Build on cognitive maturity
- Focus on fostering positive relationships
- Highlight support mechanisms

However much the topics of self-harm and suicide are discussed, it is still very less. This is a problem demanding the urgent attention of the adults who surround the child, actively engaging in intervening in the child's thought process and plans to inflict any harm or injury to the self. Environment, people and media—all play significant contributory roles which need to have 'sensitivity' as their key word.

# Fortis Healthcare Limited

Fortis Healthcare Limited is a leading integrated healthcare delivery service provider in India. The healthcare verticals of the company primarily comprise hospitals, diagnostics and day care specialty facilities. Currently, the company operates its healthcare delivery services in India, Dubai, Mauritius and Sri Lanka with 45 healthcare facilities (including projects under development), approximately 10,000 potential beds and over 346 diagnostic centres.

# Fortis School Mental Health Program

The Fortis School Mental Health Program since its inception has been extending its services to students, teachers, parents and all other stakeholders involved in a student's life. It is a platform that promotes psychosocial health and well-being of schoolchildren through the provision of therapeutic, preventive and rehabilitative services. The program focuses on enhancing life skills of children and adolescents to help them cope effectively with the challenges of life and preparing them for most contingencies.

The program has a dual focus—a strong impetus on clinical aspects of working with the young population of the country, as well as building resilience through workshops and seminars. The development of life skills is integral to work done through the Fortis Pro-Social Peer Moderator Program. Also, skill acquisition and knowledge development are the cornerstones of the Fortis School Counsellor Forum.

The multi-disciplinary team of experts comprising psychiatrists, clinical psychologists, counselling psychologists, psychodynamic psychotherapists, special educators, occupational therapists, art-based therapists and sport psychologists, work collaboratively to ensure the best service provision under one roof for all children and adolescents' mental health needs.

# References

American Psychiatric Association, *Diagnostic and Statistical Manual of Mental Disorders*, 5th ed., Arlington, VA, American Psychiatric Association, 2013.

Antony, M.M., Roth, D., Swinson, R.P., Huta, V., & Devins, G.M., 'Illness intrusiveness in individuals with panic disorder, obsessive-compulsive disorder, or social phobia', *J Nerv Ment Dis, 186*, pp. 311–15, 1998.

Bellack, H.S. & Hersen, M., *Comprehensive Clinical Psychology*, Vol. 5, Elseiver, 2000.

Danserau, V., & Bouchard, G., 'Le trouble obsessif-compulsif chez les enfants: quel est le role de l' enseignant? (OCD in children: what is the role of the teacher?)', 2005.

Geller, D.A., Biederman, J., Jones, J., Shapiro, S., Schwartz, S., & Park, K.S., 'Obsessive-compulsive disorder in children and adolescents: a review', *Harvard Review Psychiatry, 5*, pp. 260–73, 1998.

Gini, G. & Pozolli, T., 'Association between bullying and psychosomatic problems: A meta analysis', *Pediatrics, 123* (3), pp. 1059-65. doi: 10.1542/peds, 2008–1215), 2009.

Griez, E.J.L., Faravelli, C., Nutt, D., & Zohar, D., *Anxiety Disorders: An Introduction to Clinical Management and Research*, John Wiley & Sons, 2001.

Kase, L., & Ledley, D. R., *The Wiley Concise Guides to Mental Health: Anxiety Disorders*, John Wiley & Sons, 2007.

Kessler, R.C., McGonagle, K.A., Zhao, S., Nelson, C.B., Hughes, M., Eshleman, S., Wittchen, H.U., & Kendler, K.S., 'Lifetime and 12-month prevalence of DSM-III-R psychiatric disorders in the United States: Results from the National Comorbidity Survey', *Arch Gen Psychiatry, 51*, pp. 8–19, 1994.

Khanna, S., Gururaj, G., & Sriram, T.G., 'Epidemiology of obsessive-compulsive disorder in India', presented at the first International Obsessive-

Compulsive Disorder Congress, 2009.

Lewinsohn, P.M., Klein, D.N. & Seeley, J.R., 'Bipolar disorders in a community sample of older adolescents: prevalence, phenomenology, comorbidity and course', *Journal of the American Academy of Child and Adolescent Psychiatry, 34*, pp. 454–63, 1995.

Malhi, P. & Singhi, P., 'Spectrum of attention deficit hyperactivity disorders in children among referrals to psychology services', *Indian Pediatrics, 37 (11)*, pp. 1256–60, 2000.

Merikangas, K.R., Jin, R., He, J.P., Kessler, R.C., Lee, S., Sampson, N.A., Viana, M.C., Andrade, L.H., Hu, C., Karam, E.G., Ladea, M., Medina-Mora, M.E., Ono, Y., Posada-Villa, J., Sagar, R., Wells, J.E., Zarkov, Z., 'Prevalence and Correlates of Bipolar Spectrum Disorder in the World Mental Health Survey Initiative', *Archives of General Psychiatry, 68*(3), pp. 241–51, doi:10.1001/archgenpsychiatry.2011.12.

Mupalla, S.C. (n.d.), retrieved from http://www.medindia.net/news/healthinfocus/world-mental-health-day-2010-75134-1.htm

Name.org. (n.d.), retrieved from https://www.nami.org/Learn-More/Mental-Health-Conditions/Bipolar-Disorder

National Institute of Mental Health, 'Transforming the understanding and treatment of mental illnesses', 2013.

nimh.nih.gov. (n.d.), retrieved from http://www.nimh.nih.gov/health/publications/bipolar-disorder-in-children-and-teens-easy-to-read/index.shtml

nimh.nih.gov. (n.d.), retrieved from http://www.nimh.nih.gov/health/publications/bipolar-disorder-in-children-and-adolescents/index.shtml

nimh.nih.gov. (n.d.), retrieved from http://www.nimh.nih.gov/health/publications/anxiety-disorders-in-children-and-adolescents/index.shtml

Nurnberger Jr., J.I., & Foroud, T., 'Genetics of bipolar affective disorder', *Curr Psychiatry Rep, 2(2)*, pp. 147–157, 2000.

Overbeek, T., Vermetten, E., & Griez, E. J. L., 'Epidemiology of anxiety disorders', in Griez, E. J. L., Faravelli, C., Nutt, D., & Zohar, D., *Anxiety Disorders: An Introduction to Clinical Management and Research*, John Wiley & Sons, 2001.

Porter, R.S. & Kaplan, J. L., *The Merck Manual of Diagnosis and Therapy* (19th ed.), Merck Publishing, 2011.

Pravin, D., Rajkumar, R.P., Prabhuswamy, M.Y., Srinath, S., Girimaji, S., & Shashadri, S.P., 'Course and outcome of bipolar affective disorder in children', *Journal of Indian Association for Child and Adolescent Mental Health, 5(2)*, 2011.

Reddy, Y.C., Srinath, S., Prakash, H.M,, Girimaji, S.C., Sheshadri, S.P., &

Khanna, S., 'A follow-up study of juvenile obsessive-compulsive disorder from India', *Acta Psychiatrica Scandinavica, 107,* pp. 457–64, 2003.

Regier, D.A., Narrow, W.E., Rae, D.S., Manderscheid, R.W., Locke, B.Z., Goodwin, F.K., 'The de facto mental and addictive disorders service system. Epidemiologic Catchment Area prospective 1-year prevalence rates of disorders and services', *Archives of General Psychiatry, 50* (2), pp. 85–94, 1993.

Rikert, V.I. & Jay, M.S., 'Psychosomatic disorders: the approach', *Pediatrics in Review, 15 (11),* pp. 448–54, 1994.

Rutter, M., Bishop, D., Pine, D., Scott, S., Stevenson, J., Taylor, E., & Thapar, A., *Rutter's Child and Adolescent Psychiatry,* Blackwell Publishing Inc., 2008.

Saddock, B.J., Saddock, V.A. & Ruiz, P., *Kaplan and Saddock's synopsis of psychiatry,* 11$^{th}$ ed., Wolters Kluwer, 2015.

Stoudemire A., 'Epidemiology and psychopharmacology of anxiety in medical patients', *Journal of Clinical Psychiatry, 57(7),* pp. 64–72, 73–75, 1996.

Unicef.in (n.n.), retrieved from http://www.unicef.org/india/media_2892.htm

U.S. Food and Drug Administration, retrieved from http://www.accessdata.fda.gov/scripts/sda/sdNavigation.cfm?sd=labellingdatabase

Wcd.nic.in (n.d.), retrieved from http://wcd.nic.in/childabuse.pdf

World Health Organization, *Global Burden of Disease,* Geneva, Switzerland, 1990.